THE ULTIMATE FERTILITY DIET COOKBOOK FOR COUPLES

NOURISHING RECIPES TO BOOST YOUR FERTILITY JOURNEY

BY

STEPHAINE B. HARVEY

TABLE OF CONTENTS

This comprehensive fertility diet cookbook aims to provide couples with the knowledge and tools they need to support their fertility journey through nutrition and lifestyle choices. It includes a wide range of delicious and nutrient-packed recipes, meal plans, and practical advice to help couples nourish their bodies and increase their chances of conceiving. Whether you're just starting to think about expanding your family or have been trying for a while, "THE ULTIMATE FERTILITY DIET COOKBOOK FOR COUPLES" will guide you toward a healthier and more fertility-friendly way of eating and living.

INTRODUCTION

Welcome to "The Ultimate Fertility Diet Cookbook for Couples" In the grand tapestry of life, few journeys are as profoundly rewarding and transformative as the path to parenthood. For many, this journey begins with the desire to bring a new life into the world and nurture a family.

However, for some couples, the road to parenthood may be paved with challenges. Fertility struggles can be emotionally and physically taxing, leaving individuals and partners feeling overwhelmed, frustrated, and even hopeless at times. It's during these moments of uncertainty and longing that we often seek answers and solutions.

This cookbook is a labor of love, carefully crafted to offer a glimmer of hope, a ray of guidance, and a wealth of nourishing recipes tailored to support your fertility journey. Within these pages, you will discover the incredible impact that nutrition and lifestyle choices can have on your reproductive health and overall well-being.

We believe that a journey toward parenthood should not only be about overcoming obstacles but also about fostering health, wellness, and resilience. By adopting a fertility-focused diet and lifestyle, you can empower yourselves with the knowledge and tools to enhance your chances of conceiving while nurturing your bodies and your love for one another.

In the following chapters, we will explore the foundations of a fertility diet, the importance of a fertility-friendly kitchen, the role of superfoods, and practical meal plans designed for both partners. We will delve into the significance of a holistic approach to fertility, encompassing not only what you eat but also how you live, move, and connect.

This cookbook is not just about food; it's about nourishing love—your love for each other and the love you have for the life you hope to create together. It's about embracing the journey, finding strength in unity, and savoring each step along the way.

Remember, every family's journey is unique, and there is no one-size-fits-all solution. "THE ULTIMATE FERTILITY DIET COOKBOOK FOR COUPLES" is here to be your companion, offering guidance, inspiration, and a culinary adventure as you embark on this life-changing quest. Together, let's nourish not only your bodies but also your dreams of building a loving family.

With love and hope,

Stephaine B. Harvey

WHY NUTRITION MATTERS FOR FERTILITY

Before we dive into the delicious recipes and meal plans designed to enhance your fertility, let's take a moment to explore why nutrition plays a pivotal role in your ability to conceive. Understanding the connection between what you eat and your reproductive health is the first step towards making informed choices that can positively impact your fertility journey.

The Nutrient Connection

Nutrition is the foundation of life. The food we consume provides our bodies with the essential nutrients, vitamins, minerals, and energy needed to function optimally. This includes the intricate and delicate processes involved in reproduction.

1. Hormone Balance:

Hormones are the body's messengers, and they play a central role in fertility. Proper nutrition ensures that your endocrine system, responsible for hormone production, functions smoothly. Balanced hormones are crucial for regulating the menstrual cycle, ovulation, and sperm production.

2. Egg and Sperm Health:

Both partners' reproductive cells, eggs, and sperm require specific nutrients to develop properly. Nutrient deficiencies can impact the quality and viability of these cells, affecting your chances of conception.

3. Fertility-Friendly Environment:
A nutritious diet helps create a conducive environment within the body for conception. It can reduce inflammation, oxidative stress, and other factors that may hinder fertility.

4. Maintaining a Healthy Weight:
Nutrition also plays a role in maintaining a healthy body weight. Excess body weight or extreme underweight can disrupt hormonal balance and interfere with fertility.

INFLAMMATION AND OXIDATIVE STRESS
Inflammation and oxidative stress are two factors that can significantly impact fertility. Inflammation is the body's response to injury or infection, and chronic inflammation can disrupt normal reproductive processes. Oxidative stress occurs when there is an imbalance between free radicals and antioxidants in the body, potentially damaging reproductive cells.

Fortunately, an anti-inflammatory and antioxidant-rich diet can help mitigate these effects, promoting a more fertile environment.

LIFESTYLE FACTORS

Nutrition is only one piece of the puzzle. Lifestyle factors such as physical activity, stress management, and sleep also play crucial roles in fertility. In this cookbook, we will not only explore the right foods but also provide guidance on creating a holistic approach to support your fertility journey.

In the chapters ahead, we will delve deeper into the specific nutrients, superfoods, and meal plans that can boost fertility for both partners. Remember that every couple's journey is unique, and this cookbook is designed to be a versatile resource to meet your individual needs and preferences.

So, let's embark on this culinary journey together, nourishing not only your bodies but also your hopes and dreams of starting or expanding your family.

Bon appétit!

HOW THIS COOKBOOK CAN HELP

As you embark on your fertility journey, you might wonder how this cookbook can assist you in achieving your goals. "The Ultimate Fertility Diet Cookbook for Couples" is more than just a collection of recipes; it's a comprehensive guide designed to provide you with the knowledge, tools, and practical resources needed to support your fertility and overall well-being.

1. NUTRITIONAL GUIDANCE:

This cookbook offers valuable insights into the specific nutrients and dietary choices that can enhance your fertility. You'll learn which foods are fertility-boosting powerhouses and why they matter.

2. FERTILITY MEAL PLANS:

We provide carefully crafted meal plans for both partners, making it easy to incorporate fertility-friendly foods into your daily life. These meal plans take the guesswork out of meal preparation, ensuring that you get the nutrients you need.

3. RECIPES FOR WELLNESS:

Discover a wide range of delicious and nourishing recipes tailored to support fertility. From breakfast options to snacks, dinners, and desserts, these recipes are designed to be both nutritious and enjoyable.

4. LIFESTYLE INSIGHTS:

Fertility isn't just about what you eat; it's also influenced by how you live. This cookbook delves into lifestyle factors such as exercise, stress management, and sleep, offering guidance on creating a holistic approach to fertility.

5. SPECIAL DIETARY NEEDS:

We understand that dietary preferences and restrictions vary widely. You'll find information and recipes catering to various dietary needs, including vegan, vegetarian, gluten-free, and allergy-friendly options.

6. FERTILITY RESOURCES:

Throughout the cookbook, you'll find additional resources, references, and recommendations for further reading and exploration. We want to empower you with the knowledge you need to make informed choices.

7. A JOURNEY SHARED:

This book acknowledges that the fertility journey is a shared experience between partners. We provide tips on how to communicate effectively, offer emotional support, and strengthen your bond as a couple.

8. CELEBRATING SUCCESS STORIES

Along the way, you'll encounter stories of couples who have successfully navigated their fertility challenges. These stories serve as a source of inspiration and hope.

Remember that your fertility journey is unique, and there is no one-size-fits-all solution. This cookbook is here to serve as a flexible and supportive companion, adapting to your individual needs and preferences. Whether you're just starting to think about expanding your family or have been trying for a while, this cookbook aims to empower you with the tools to nourish not only your bodies but also your dreams of building a loving family.

Let's embark on this journey together, one nourishing meal at a time, as we work toward the shared goal of bringing new life into the world and nurturing the love that brought you together.

With love and nourishment.

CHAPTER 1:

UNDERSTANDING FERTILITY

In this introductory chapter, we will delve into the core concepts surrounding fertility, providing a foundational understanding for couples on their journey to parenthood.

The Miracle Of Life

- Exploring the awe-inspiring process of conception, embryonic development, and childbirth.

- Highlighting the remarkable journey of sperm meeting egg and the formation of a new life.

The Fertility Window

- Defining the concept of a fertility window or fertility window, the period during which conception is most likely.

- Discussing the factors that influence the timing of fertility, including the menstrual cycle and ovulation.

Factors Affecting Fertility

- Investigating the multitude of factors that can impact fertility, including age, genetics, lifestyle, and health.

- Understanding how environmental factors, stress, and underlying medical conditions may play a role.

Natural vs. Assisted Conception

- Contrasting natural conception methods with assisted reproductive technologies (ART) such as in vitro fertilization (IVF).

- Providing an overview of when and how assisted conception options might be considered.

Emotional and Psychological Aspects

- Acknowledging the emotional and psychological aspects of fertility, including the desire for parenthood, expectations, and the stress that can accompany the journey.

Cultural and Societal Influences

- Exploring how cultural and societal norms and expectations can impact individuals and couples dealing with fertility challenges.

By the end of this chapter, readers will have a solid grasp of what fertility encompasses, the factors that can influence it, and the emotional and societal dimensions that often accompany this profound aspect of human existence. This understanding sets the stage for couples to navigate their fertility journey with knowledge and sensitivity.

THE BASICS OF REPRODUCTIVE HEALTH

1. ANATOMY AND PHYSIOLOGY OF REPRODUCTIVE HEALTH

Understanding the male and female reproductive systems is fundamental to grasping reproductive health.

Male Reproductive System:

- **Testes**: These are the primary male reproductive organs responsible for producing sperm and testosterone.
- **Epididymis**: A coiled tube where sperm mature and are stored.
- **Vas Deferens**: Tubes that transport sperm from the epididymis to the urethra during ejaculation.
- **Urethra**: The tube that carries both urine and semen out of the body.
- **Accessory Glands:** These include the seminal vesicles, prostate gland, and bulbourethral glands, which contribute fluids to semen.

Female Reproductive System:

- **Ovaries**: These organs produce eggs (ova) and female sex hormones like estrogen and progesterone.
- **Fallopian Tubes:** Tubes that transport eggs from the ovaries to the uterus and serve as the site of fertilization.
- **Uterus**: The womb where a fertilized egg implants and grows during pregnancy.

- **Cervix**: The lower part of the uterus that connects to the vagina.
- **Vagina**: The birth canal and the site of sperm deposition during intercourse.

2. HORMONES AND REGULATION

Hormones play a crucial role in regulating the reproductive systems in both men and women.

Male Hormones:

- **Testosterone**: The primary male sex hormone responsible for sperm production, muscle and bone development, and secondary sexual characteristics.
- **Follicle-Stimulating Hormone (FSH) and Luteinizing Hormone (LH):** These hormones from the pituitary gland regulate testicular function and sperm production.

Female Hormones:

- **Estrogen**: The main female sex hormone responsible for regulating the menstrual cycle, promoting egg development, and maintaining the uterine lining.
- **Progesterone**: Prepares the uterine lining for potential pregnancy and supports early pregnancy.

3. OVULATION AND MENSTRUATION

The menstrual cycle is a key aspect of reproductive health in women.

- **Menstrual Cycle Phases:** The cycle is divided into phases, including menstruation, the follicular phase (leading up to ovulation), and the luteal phase (after ovulation).
- **Ovulation:** The release of a mature egg from the ovaries into the fallopian tubes, typically occurring midway through the menstrual cycle.
- **Menstruation:** The shedding of the uterine lining if pregnancy does not occur.

Understanding these basics is crucial for individuals and couples interested in family planning and maintaining reproductive health. It enables them to make informed decisions about contraception, fertility, and overall well-being.

COMMON FERTILITY CHALLENGES

1. INFERTILITY DEFINED:

- **Primary Infertility**: Couples who have not achieved a pregnancy after at least one year of regular, unprotected intercourse.

- **Secondary Infertility**: Couples who have previously had a successful pregnancy but are now struggling to conceive again.

2. CAUSES OF INFERTILITY:

- **Advanced Age:** Fertility tends to decline with age, especially after the age of 35 for women.

- **Medical Conditions**: Conditions like polycystic ovary syndrome (PCOS), endometriosis, fibroids, and thyroid disorders can impact fertility.

- **Sexual Dysfunction**: Problems with sexual function or performance can hinder conception.

- **Low Sperm Count and Quality**: In men, issues with sperm production, motility, or morphology can lead to infertility.

- **Tubal Blockages:** Blockages or damage to the fallopian tubes can prevent the egg from reaching the uterus or sperm from reaching the egg.

- **Unexplained Infertility:** In some cases, no specific cause of infertility can be identified, despite extensive testing.

3. RECURRENT PREGNANCY LOSS:

- Some couples may experience the heartache of recurrent miscarriages (usually defined as three or more consecutive pregnancy losses). This can have both physical and emotional implications.

Male And Female Factors:

- **Female Factors**: Conditions like PCOS, endometriosis, blocked fallopian tubes, and hormonal imbalances can impact a woman's fertility.
- **Male Factors**: Low sperm count, poor sperm motility, erectile dysfunction, and genetic issues can affect male fertility.

5. LIFESTYLE AND ENVIRONMENTAL FACTORS:

- **Smoking and Alcohol**: Tobacco and excessive alcohol consumption can negatively affect fertility.
- **Obesity**: Being overweight or obese can disrupt hormonal balance and reduce fertility.
- **Stress**: High levels of stress can interfere with the menstrual cycle and ovulation.
- **Environmental Toxins**: Exposure to certain chemicals, pesticides, and pollutants may affect fertility.

6. EMOTIONAL TOLL:

- Coping with fertility challenges can be emotionally challenging and stressful for both individuals and couples. The emotional toll of infertility is significant and should not be underestimated.

Understanding these common fertility challenges is essential for couples who are trying to conceive. It enables them to seek appropriate medical advice, explore treatment options, and access emotional support as they navigate their fertility journey.

CHAPTER 2:

THE FERTILITY-FRIENDLY KITCHEN

In this chapter, we will transform your kitchen into a fertility-friendly haven, where you'll find the tools, ingredients, and strategies to support your journey toward parenthood.

- **ORGANIZING YOUR FERTILITY KITCHEN**

-**Pantry Essentials**: Stocking your pantry with fertility-enhancing staples like whole grains, legumes, and healthy fats.

-**Refrigerator and Freezer Must-Haves:** Identifying fertility-friendly foods to keep on hand for quick and nutritious meals.

-**Food Storage and Organization**: Tips for keeping your ingredients fresh and accessible.

- **MEAL PLANNING FOR FERTILITY SUCCESS**

-**Weekly Meal Planning**: The benefits of planning your meals in advance and how to create a fertility-focused meal plan.

-**Grocery Shopping for Fertility**: Guidance on navigating the grocery store to make healthy and informed choices.

-**Budget-Friendly Fertility Meals:** Strategies for maintaining a fertility-friendly diet without breaking the bank.

- **PREPARING YOUR FERTILITY-FRIENDLY KITCHEN**

-**Cookware and Utensils**: Choosing the right cookware and utensils for nutrient retention.

-**Safe Food Handling**: Proper food handling practices to minimize foodborne illnesses and maximize food safety.

-**Mindful Cooking**: Techniques to preserve the nutritional value of your ingredients during the cooking process.

- **READING LABELS AND MAKING INFORMED CHOICES**

- **Understanding Food Labels**: Deciphering food labels to identify ingredients that may affect fertility, such as excessive sugars, artificial additives, and preservatives.

- **Making Informed Choices**: Tips for selecting fertility-friendly packaged foods and understanding food marketing tactics.

- **SPECIAL DIETARY CONSIDERATIONS**

-**Fertility and Dietary Restrictions**: How to adapt your fertility-friendly kitchen for specific dietary needs, such as vegetarian, vegan, or gluten-free diets.

-**Allergies and Sensitivities**: Managing food allergies and sensitivities while maintaining a fertility-focused diet.

FERTILITY MEAL PREP AND PLANNING

-**Batch Cooking:** Streamlining your meal prep with batch cooking techniques for busy days.

-**Meal Planning Apps and Tools**: Utilizing technology to simplify meal planning and shopping.

-**Creating Balanced Fertility Meals**: Strategies for building balanced and nutritious meals to support your reproductive health.

By the end of this chapter, you will have the knowledge and tools to create a well-organized, fertility-friendly kitchen that supports your dietary needs on your journey to parenthood. You'll also be equipped with meal planning and preparation skills to make nourishing meals a seamless part of your daily routine.

STOCKING YOUR PANTRY

Your pantry is the heart of your fertility-friendly kitchen. Stocking it with the right ingredients will ensure that you have the building blocks for nutritious and balanced meals that support your reproductive health.

- **<u>Whole Grains:</u>**

-**Brown Rice:** Rich in fiber and nutrients, it's a versatile base for many dishes.

-**Quinoa**: A complete protein source and excellent source of nutrients.

-**Oats**: High in fiber and can be used in breakfast options like oatmeal or granola.

- **<u>Legumes:</u>**

-**Lentils**: Packed with protein and iron, they can be used in soups, stews, and salads.

-**Chickpeas**: A good source of protein and fiber, ideal for making hummus or adding to salads.

-**Black Beans**: Rich in folate and fiber, great for Mexican-inspired dishes.

- **<u>Healthy Fats:</u>**

-**Olive Oil**: A heart-healthy fat for sautéing and dressings.

-**Nuts and Seeds:** Almonds, walnuts, chia seeds, and flaxseeds provide essential fatty acids.

-**Avocado**: A nutrient-dense source of healthy fats.

- **Canned Goods:**

-**Canned Tomatoes**: Perfect for making pasta sauces and soups.

-**Canned Salmon and Sardines**: Rich in omega-3 fatty acids and great for salads and sandwiches.

-**Canned Beans:** Convenient for adding protein and fiber to various dishes.

- **Herbs and Spices:**

- **Turmeric**: Known for its anti-inflammatory properties.

-**Cinnamon**: Adds flavor without added sugar, ideal for oatmeal and smoothies.

-**Ginger**: Adds a unique taste and is great for digestive health.

- **Whole-Grain Pasta and Flour:**

-**Whole-Grain Pasta:** A healthier alternative to regular pasta.

- **Whole-Grain Flour:** Useful for baking fertility-friendly treats.

- **Dried Fruits:**

-**Dried Apricots and Dates**: Natural sweeteners for recipes.

-**Raisins**: Ideal for adding natural sweetness to oatmeal or yogurt.

- **<u>Nut Butter:</u>**

-**Almond or Peanut Butter**: Provides protein and healthy fats for snacks or spreads.

- **<u>Vinegars and Condiments:</u>**

-**Balsamic Vinegar**: For salad dressings and marinades.
-**Soy Sauce or Tamari**: For flavoring dishes.
-**Dijon Mustard**: Adds depth to salad dressings.

- **<u>Herbs and Spices:</u>**

- **Sea Salt**: Use in moderation for flavor.
- **Black Pepper**: Enhances the taste of dishes.
- **Dried Herbs:** Such as basil, thyme, and oregano for seasoning.

Remember to check expiration dates, and periodically review your pantry to ensure freshness. Stocking your pantry with these items sets the stage for creating nourishing and fertility-boosting meals.

ESSENTIAL KITCHEN TOOLS

To create a fertility-friendly kitchen that supports your journey, you'll need the right tools to prepare and cook your meals efficiently. Here are essential kitchen tools to consider:

- **Chef's Knife:**
A high-quality chef's knife is your kitchen workhorse, suitable for chopping, slicing, and dicing a variety of ingredients.

- **Cutting Board**:
Invest in a durable, easy-to-clean cutting board to protect your countertops and ensure food safety.

- **Measuring Cups and Spoons:**
Accurate measurements are crucial for following recipes and portion control.

- **Mixing Bowls:**
Assortment of mixing bowls in different sizes for mixing ingredients, marinating, and food prep.

- **Pots and Pans:**
A set of high-quality pots and pans, including a saucepan, skillet, and stockpot, will cover most cooking needs.

- **Baking Sheets and Pans:**

For roasting vegetables, baking fertility-friendly treats, and making sheet pan meals.

- **Blender or Food Processor:**

Great for making smoothies, soups, and purees. A food processor is versatile for chopping and mixing.

- **Grater and Zester:**

For grating vegetables, fruits, and adding zest to dishes for flavor.

- **Vegetable Peeler:**

A sharp vegetable peeler makes it easier to peel and prepare vegetables and fruits.

- **Colander or Strainer:**

For draining pasta, rinsing vegetables, and more.

- **Thermometer:**

An instant-read thermometer ensures that meats and other foods are cooked to a safe temperature.

- **Oven Mitts and Pot Holders:**

Protect your hands and surfaces while handling hot cookware.

- **Kitchen Timer:**

A timer helps you keep track of cooking times and prevent overcooking.

- **Food Scale:**

Useful for precise measurements, especially for portion control.

- **Can Opener:**

For opening canned goods like beans and tomatoes.

- **Salad Spinner:**

Efficiently wash and dry greens and herbs for salads.

- **Wooden Spoons and Spatulas:**

Non-reactive utensils for stirring and flipping in cookware.

18. Tongs:
Versatile for flipping, turning, and serving various foods.

19. Whisk:
For mixing, whipping, and emulsifying ingredients in recipes.

20. Kitchen Gadgets:
Consider specialty tools like a citrus juicer, garlic press, or egg timer if you frequently use these ingredients.

Having these essential kitchen tools at your disposal will make meal preparation more convenient and enjoyable, ensuring that you can easily create fertility-boosting dishes as part of your fertility journey.

CHAPTER 3:

THE FOUNDATIONS OF A FERTILITY DIET

In this chapter, we'll explore the core principles and food groups that form the foundation of a fertility-boosting diet. These guidelines will help you make informed choices to support your reproductive health and increase your chances of conception.

THE FERTILITY-BOOSTING FOOD GROUPS

- **Leafy Greens and Vegetables:**

Discover the importance of greens like spinach and broccoli, and colorful vegetables rich in vitamins and antioxidants.

- **Whole Grains:**

Explore the benefits of whole grains like quinoa, brown rice, and oats for hormone balance and sustained energy.

- **Lean Proteins:**

Understand the significance of lean protein sources such as poultry, fish, and plant-based proteins in supporting fertility.

- **Healthy Fats:**

Learn about the role of healthy fats from sources like avocados, nuts, and olive oil in reproductive health.

- **Fruits and Berries:**

Explore the wide array of fruits and berries that provide essential vitamins and antioxidants.

NUTRIENT DENSITY AND BALANCE

The Importance of Nutrient Density:

Understand why choosing nutrient-dense foods is crucial for fertility.

Balancing Macronutrients:

Learn how to create balanced meals that include carbohydrates, proteins, and fats in the right proportions.

MINDFUL EATING AND PORTION CONTROL

Mindful Eating Practices:

Discover techniques for mindful eating that can support your fertility journey.

Portion Control:

Understand the significance of portion control for maintaining a healthy weight and hormonal balance.

THE ROLE OF HYDRATION

Hydration and Fertility:

Learn how staying well-hydrated can positively affect reproductive health.

Best Beverage Choices:
Explore the beverages that are ideal for fertility and those to consume in moderation.

COOKING TECHNIQUES FOR NUTRIENT RETENTION

Cooking Methods:
Understand how different cooking methods can affect the nutritional content of your food.

Minimizing Nutrient Loss:
Learn tips and techniques to preserve the maximum nutrients in your meals.

SPECIAL CONSIDERATIONS

Fertility and Dietary Restrictions:
Explore how to adapt the foundations of a fertility diet to specific dietary needs, such as vegetarian, vegan, or gluten-free diets.

Allergies And Sensitivities:
Manage food allergies and sensitivities while maintaining a fertility-focused diet.

By the end of this chapter, you will have a solid understanding of the fundamental principles of a fertility diet. You'll be equipped with the knowledge needed to make informed food choices, create balanced meals, and incorporate fertility-boosting ingredients into your daily diet to support your reproductive health.

1. NUTRIENT-RICH FOODS FOR BOTH PARTNERS

Incorporating nutrient-rich foods into your diet can benefit both partners on their fertility journey. Here are some fertility-boosting foods for both men and women:

- **LEAFY GREENS:**

Benefits for Women:

Spinach, kale, and collard greens are rich in folate, a crucial nutrient for healthy egg development.

Benefits for Men:

These greens are packed with antioxidants that help protect sperm from damage.

- **BERRIES:**

Benefits for Women:

Berries like blueberries and strawberries are high in antioxidants, which can help improve egg quality.

Benefits for Men:

Antioxidants in berries also support sperm health and motility.

- **FATTY FISH:**

<u>Benefits for Women:</u>

Salmon, mackerel, and sardines are excellent sources of omega-3 fatty acids, which can regulate hormones and promote reproductive health.

<u>Benefits for Men:</u>

Omega-3s support sperm quality and motility.

- **WHOLE GRAINS:**

<u>Benefits for Women:</u>

Whole grains like quinoa and brown rice provide complex carbohydrates and fiber, helping to regulate blood sugar levels and hormone balance.

<u>Benefits for Men:</u>

These grains provide energy and nutrients essential for sperm production.

- **LEAN PROTEIN:**

<u>Benefits for Women:</u>

Lean protein sources like chicken and tofu supply amino acids that support egg health.

<u>Benefits for Men:</u>

Protein is essential for building healthy sperm.

- **NUTS AND SEEDS:**

<u>Benefits for Women:</u>

Almonds, walnuts, and chia seeds are rich in healthy fats and antioxidants that can support reproductive health.

<u>Benefits for Men:</u>

Nuts and seeds provide essential nutrients for sperm production and quality.

- **AVOCADO:**

<u>Benefits for Women:</u>

Avocado's healthy fats can help with hormone regulation.

<u>Benefits for Men:</u>

The same fats support sperm health and motility.

- **BEANS AND LEGUMES:**

<u>Benefits for Women:</u>

Lentils and chickpeas are excellent sources of plant-based protein and iron, important for fertility.

<u>Benefits for Men:</u>

These foods provide essential nutrients for sperm health.

- **DAIRY OR DAIRY ALTERNATIVES:**

<u>Benefits for Women:</u>

Dairy products offer calcium and vitamin D, important for reproductive health.

<u>Benefits for Men:</u>

Calcium supports sperm function.

- **EGGS:**

Benefits for Women:

Eggs provide high-quality protein and essential vitamins like B12 and choline, important for fertility.

Benefits for Men:

Eggs contain nutrients that support sperm production.

Including these nutrient-rich foods in both partners' diets can contribute to improved reproductive health and increase the chances of a successful conception. Remember that a balanced and varied diet is key, and it's advisable to consult with a healthcare professional or registered dietitian for personalized dietary guidance on your fertility journey.

2. HYDRATION AND FERTILITY

Proper hydration is crucial for overall health, including reproductive health. Here's how staying well-hydrated can positively affect fertility for both partners:

- **CERVICAL MUCUS QUALITY:**

Hydration plays a role in cervical mucus production. Cervical mucus is essential for sperm transport and survival within the female reproductive tract.

Being well-hydrated can lead to more abundant and fertile-quality cervical mucus, which can facilitate sperm movement towards the egg.

- **HORMONE REGULATION:**

Dehydration can disrupt hormonal balance, including the hormones that regulate the menstrual cycle in women and sperm production in men.

Proper hydration helps maintain hormonal equilibrium, which is essential for reproductive health.

- **TEMPERATURE REGULATION:**

Dehydration can lead to an increase in body temperature. Elevated body temperature can negatively impact sperm production and egg quality.

Staying hydrated helps regulate body temperature, which is particularly crucial for men and their sperm production.

- **BLOOD FLOW:**

Proper hydration supports healthy blood circulation. This is vital for the delivery of nutrients and oxygen to reproductive organs.

Adequate blood flow to the reproductive organs ensures their optimal function.

- **GENERAL WELL-BEING:**

Dehydration can lead to fatigue, irritability, and stress, all of which can impact sexual health and desire.

Being well-hydrated promotes overall well-being and a more positive attitude towards conception.

TIPS FOR STAYING HYDRATED:
1. **Drink Water Regularly:** Aim for at least 8 glasses (about 2 liters) of water per day. Adjust this based on your individual needs and activity level.

2. **Monitor Urine Color:** Pale yellow urine is a good indicator of proper hydration. Dark yellow or amber urine may signal dehydration.

3. **Incorporate Hydrating Foods**: Consume foods with high water content, such as fruits (watermelon, cucumber) and vegetables (lettuce, celery).

4. **Limit Dehydrating Beverages**: Reduce or avoid beverages like caffeinated drinks and alcohol, which can contribute to dehydration.

5. **Stay Hydrated During Exercise**: If you're physically active, drink water before, during, and after exercise to replace fluids lost through sweat.

6. **Listen to Your Body:** Thirst is a clear signal that your body needs hydration. Don't ignore it.

Remember that individual hydration needs can vary, so it's essential to pay attention to your body's signals and adjust your fluid intake accordingly. Ensuring proper hydration is a simple yet effective step toward supporting your fertility and overall health.

CHAPTER 4:

PLANNING MEALS WITH FERTILITY IN MIND

In this chapter, we'll dive into the art of meal planning specifically tailored to boost fertility. You'll learn how to create well-balanced, nourishing meals that support reproductive health for both partners.

➤ BREAKFAST BOOSTERS FOR FERTILITY

Breakfast is a crucial meal for providing energy and essential nutrients to kickstart your day and support fertility. Here are some breakfast boosters tailored for reproductive health for both partners:

• FOLATE-RICH FOODS:

For Women:
Start your day with folate-rich foods like spinach and kale omelets or avocado toast. Folate is essential for healthy egg development.

For Men:
Include foods like lentils and black beans, which provide folate that supports sperm health.

- **OMEGA-3 FATTY ACIDS:**

<u>**For Women:**</u>

Opt for a breakfast smoothie with chia seeds or flaxseed, both high in omega-3s that can help regulate hormones.

<u>**For Men:**</u>

Consider a serving of fatty fish like salmon or sardines to support sperm quality.

- **PROTEIN-PACKED OPTIONS:**

<u>**For Women:**</u>

Greek yogurt with berries and nuts or a vegetable and egg scramble provide protein and essential nutrients.

<u>**For Men:**</u>

Include lean protein sources like turkey or tofu to support sperm production.

- **FIBER-RICH CHOICES:**

<u>**For Women:**</u>

Whole-grain oatmeal topped with fruits and nuts is not only nutritious but also provides fiber for hormone balance.

<u>**For Men:**</u>

Incorporate whole-grain toast or cereal to boost fiber intake, which can aid in overall health.

- **ANTIOXIDANT-RICH FRUITS:**

For Women:

Berries like blueberries and strawberries are rich in antioxidants that can help improve egg quality.

For Men:

Citrus fruits like oranges and grapefruits provide vitamin C, which supports sperm health.

- **DAIRY OR DAIRY ALTERNATIVES:**

For Women:

Greek yogurt or fortified dairy alternatives like almond milk provide calcium and vitamin D for reproductive health.

For Men:

Consider a serving of low-fat dairy or fortified plant-based milk to support sperm function.

- **HYDRATION:**

For Both Partners:

Start your day with a glass of water to stay well-hydrated, which is essential for overall health and fertility.

- **BREAKFAST SMOOTHIES:**

For Both Partners:

Customize your smoothies with fertility-boosting ingredients like spinach, berries, flaxseeds, and protein powder for a nutrient-packed morning option.

Remember to personalize your breakfast choices to meet your specific dietary preferences and nutritional needs. A well-rounded and nutritious breakfast sets the tone for a day of balanced eating that supports reproductive health.

➢ LUNCH FOR LOVE

Lunch is an excellent opportunity to fuel your body with fertility-boosting nutrients. Here are some lunch ideas that promote reproductive health for both partners:

- **LEAFY GREEN SALADS:**

For Women:

A spinach or kale salad with colorful vegetables, chickpeas, and a vinaigrette dressing provides folate, antioxidants, and fiber.

For Men:

Add lean protein like grilled chicken or tofu to support sperm health.

- **QUINOA BOWLS:**

For Both Partners:

Create quinoa bowls with a variety of veggies, avocado, and a source of lean protein like beans or salmon. Quinoa is rich in protein and nutrients.

- **WHOLE-GRAIN WRAPS:**

For Women:

Make a whole-grain wrap with hummus, roasted veggies, and leafy greens for a fiber-rich option.

For Men:

Consider a turkey or chicken wrap with plenty of colorful veggies for added antioxidants.

- **LENTIL SOUP:**

For Both Partners:

Lentil soup is rich in folate, fiber, and protein. Pair it with a side salad for a balanced meal.

- **TUNA OR SALMON SALAD:**

For Women:

Prepare a tuna or salmon salad with mixed greens and whole-grain crackers for omega-3 fatty acids and protein.

For Men:

Include plenty of vegetables in the salad to boost nutrient intake.

- **QUICHE OR FRITTATA:**

For Both Partners:

A vegetable-packed quiche or frittata made with eggs and low-fat cheese provides protein and essential vitamins.

- **BUDDHA BOWLS:**

For Women:

Create a Buddha bowl with brown rice, roasted sweet potatoes, chickpeas, and tahini dressing for a nutrient-dense lunch.

For Men:

Add lean protein like grilled shrimp or tofu for extra support.

- **FRUIT SALAD:**

For Both Partners:

A colorful fruit salad with a variety of fruits like berries, oranges, and kiwi provides antioxidants and essential vitamins.

- **HYDRATION:**

For Both Partners:

Remember to stay hydrated with water or herbal teas throughout the day to support overall health and fertility.

LEFTOVERS FROM DINNER:

For Both Partners:

Don't forget the convenience of leftovers from a fertility-friendly dinner. Reheat and enjoy a nutritious lunch the next day.

Customize these lunch options to suit your tastes and dietary preferences. A balanced and nutrient-rich lunch can provide the energy and essential nutrients needed to support reproductive health for both partners on their fertility journey.

➢ DINNERS FOR TWO

Dinner is a wonderful opportunity for couples to share a nourishing meal together that supports their fertility. Here are some dinner ideas tailored for reproductive health:

- **GRILLED SALMON WITH QUINOA AND ROASTED VEGETABLES:**
  - Salmon is rich in omega-3 fatty acids, which can benefit both partners' fertility.
  - Quinoa provides protein and essential nutrients, and roasted vegetables add fiber and antioxidants.

- **VEGETABLE STIR-FRY WITH TOFU OR LEAN CHICKEN:**
  - A stir-fry loaded with colorful vegetables, tofu, or lean chicken offers a balanced mix of nutrients and proteins.
  - The variety of veggies provides essential vitamins and minerals for reproductive health.

- **LENTIL AND VEGETABLE CURRY:**
  - Lentils are an excellent source of plant-based protein and folate.

- A vegetable curry made with a variety of spices adds flavor and antioxidants.

- **WHOLE-GRAIN PASTA WITH TOMATO SAUCE AND LEAN GROUND TURKEY:**
- Whole-grain pasta provides complex carbohydrates and fiber.
- Lean ground turkey offers protein, while tomato sauce provides vitamins and lycopene, which can support reproductive health.

- **QUINOA-STUFFED BELL PEPPERS:**
- Bell peppers stuffed with quinoa, black beans, and veggies create a well-rounded meal.
- Quinoa and beans provide protein and fiber, while the peppers offer essential vitamins.

- **BAKED SWEET POTATO WITH BLACK BEAN CHILI:**
- Sweet potatoes are rich in beta-carotene, a precursor to vitamin A.
- Black bean chili is packed with protein and fiber, supporting fertility for both partners.

- **GRILLED VEGETABLE AND CHICKPEA SALAD:**
- A salad with grilled vegetables, chickpeas, and a lemon-tahini dressing is both satisfying and nutritious.

- Chickpeas add protein and fiber, while grilled veggies provide vitamins and antioxidants.

- **HOMEMADE SUSHI ROLLS:**
- Make sushi rolls at home with avocado, cucumber, and salmon or tofu.
  - Salmon and tofu provide essential nutrients for reproductive health.

- **PORTOBELLO MUSHROOM BURGERS:**
- Portobello mushroom caps make delicious burger patties when grilled or roasted.
  - Serve them on whole-grain buns with plenty of veggies and a side salad.

- **HYDRATION:**
- Don't forget to accompany your meal with water or fertility-friendly beverages to stay hydrated.

These dinner ideas offer a variety of nutrient-rich options to support reproductive health for both partners. Cooking and sharing a wholesome meal together can also strengthen the bond between couples as they embark on their fertility journey.

➤ **SNACKS AND TREATS**

Snacks and Treats for Fertility and Enjoyment.

Between meals, it's essential to have satisfying snacks that not only curb cravings but also provide nutrients that support fertility. Here are some snack and treat ideas that can be enjoyed by both partners:

- **GREEK YOGURT WITH BERRIES:**
  - Greek yogurt is a protein-rich snack that also provides calcium and probiotics.
  - Top it with fresh berries for antioxidants and natural sweetness.

- **MIXED NUTS AND SEEDS:**
  - A handful of mixed nuts (like almonds, walnuts, and pistachios) and seeds (like chia and flax) offer healthy fats, protein, and fertility-friendly nutrients.

- **HUMMUS WITH VEGETABLE STICKS:**
  - Hummus made from chickpeas provides protein and fiber.
  - Dip carrot, cucumber, and bell pepper sticks for a crunchy, nutrient-rich snack.

- **AVOCADO TOAST:**
  - Whole-grain toast with mashed avocado and a sprinkle of sesame seeds or red pepper flakes offers healthy fats and fiber.

- **DARK CHOCOLATE AND ALMONDS:**
- Dark chocolate (with at least 70% cocoa) and almonds provide antioxidants and can satisfy sweet cravings in moderation.

- **SMOOTHIE BOWLS:**
- Create smoothie bowls with blended fruits, Greek yogurt, and toppings like granola, nuts, and seeds for a filling and nutritious treat.

- **POPCORN WITH NUTRITIONAL YEAST:**
- Air-popped popcorn seasoned with nutritional yeast adds a cheesy flavor and extra vitamins and minerals.

- **SLICED APPLES WITH PEANUT BUTTER:**
- Apples offer fiber and vitamins, while peanut butter provides protein and healthy fats.

- **CHIA PUDDING:**
- Chia seeds soaked in almond milk with a touch of honey and fresh berries create a delicious and nutrient-rich pudding.

- **FRUIT SALAD WITH MINT:**
- A fruit salad with a sprig of fresh mint can be a refreshing and hydrating snack option.

- **HERBAL TEAS:**
- Enjoy caffeine-free herbal teas like chamomile or peppermint for a soothing and hydrating beverage.

- **FROZEN YOGURT BITES:**
- Freeze Greek yogurt in small portions with added berries or honey for a cool and nutritious treat.

Remember that portion control is essential when enjoying snacks and treats. While these options can be both delicious and supportive of fertility, moderation is key. It's also a good idea to consult with a healthcare professional or registered dietitian for personalized guidance on your fertility journey, including snack choices that align with your specific needs and preferences.

➢ **BEVERAGES**

Here are some fertility-friendly beverage options that can support your reproductive health:

- **WATER:**
- Staying well-hydrated is essential for overall health and fertility. Aim to drink plenty of plain water throughout the day.

- **HERBAL TEAS:**

- Certain herbal teas, such as chamomile, peppermint, and raspberry leaf tea, are caffeine-free and can promote relaxation and balance.

- **GREEN TEA:**

-Green tea is a source of antioxidants and may have potential fertility benefits. However, it contains caffeine, so consume it in moderation.

- **FERTILITY SMOOTHIES:**

- Create smoothies with fertility-boosting ingredients like spinach, berries, Greek yogurt, and a sprinkle of flaxseeds or chia seeds.

- **FERTILITY-FRIENDLY MOCKTAILS:**

- Create mocktails using ingredients like fruit juices, sparkling water, and herbs. For example, a berry and mint spritzer can be a refreshing option.

- **COCONUT WATER:**

- Coconut water is a hydrating and electrolyte-rich beverage that can be a good choice, especially if you're active.

- **POMEGRANATE JUICE:**
  - Pomegranate juice is rich in antioxidants and may have potential fertility benefits. It can be consumed in moderation.

- **MILK ALTERNATIVES:**
  - If you're lactose intolerant or prefer plant-based options, consider almond milk, soy milk, or oat milk fortified with calcium and vitamin D.

- **PINEAPPLE JUICE:**
  - Pineapple contains bromelain, an enzyme that may have anti-inflammatory properties. Some believe it may be beneficial for fertility.

- **WATER WITH LEMON:**
  - A simple glass of water with a squeeze of fresh lemon can be a refreshing and hydrating choice.

- **FERMENTED BEVERAGES:**
  - Fermented beverages like kefir or kombucha can promote gut health, which is indirectly linked to overall well-being and fertility.

- **FERTILITY-FOCUSED HERBAL BLENDS:**
  - Some herbal blends are specifically formulated to support reproductive health. Be sure to consult with a

healthcare provider before trying any herbal supplements.

- **HYDRATION INFUSIONS:**
  - Infuse your water with slices of cucumber, strawberries, or fresh herbs like mint for added flavor.

Remember that moderation is key, especially when it comes to beverages that contain caffeine or added sugars. It's essential to maintain a balanced diet and lifestyle to support your fertility journey, and your healthcare provider can provide personalized guidance based on your specific needs and goals.

THE IMPORTANCE OF STAYING HYDRATED.
Staying hydrated is crucial for overall health and plays a significant role in supporting fertility and reproductive health. Here's why staying hydrated is so important, especially during the fertility journey:

- **HORMONAL BALANCE:**
Proper hydration helps maintain hormonal balance, which is essential for both men and women's reproductive health. Hormones like luteinizing hormone (LH) and follicle-stimulating hormone (FSH) are involved in the menstrual cycle and sperm production. Dehydration can disrupt these hormonal processes.

- **CERVICAL MUCUS PRODUCTION:**

Adequate hydration supports the production of cervical mucus. Cervical mucus changes in consistency throughout the menstrual cycle and plays a vital role in facilitating sperm transport to the egg. Dehydration can lead to thicker and less fertile cervical mucus.

- **OVULATION AND EGG QUALITY:**

For women, staying hydrated can support regular ovulation and healthy egg development. Dehydration can potentially affect the quality of eggs and interfere with the ovulation process.

- **SPERM HEALTH:**

For men, dehydration can lead to decreased sperm count and motility. Proper hydration helps ensure that sperm are abundant and capable of swimming effectively, which is crucial for fertilization.

- **UTERINE HEALTH:**

Good hydration supports the health of the uterine lining. A well-hydrated uterine lining is more conducive to embryo implantation.

- **OVERALL HEALTH:**

Hydration is essential for overall physical well-being. It helps regulate body temperature, aids digestion, and supports the circulation of nutrients and oxygen to cells throughout the body.

- **REDUCING STRESS:**

Dehydration can contribute to increased stress levels. Stress, in turn, can negatively impact fertility. Staying hydrated can help manage stress and its potential effects on reproductive health.

- **AVOIDING URINARY TRACT INFECTIONS (UTIS):**

Proper hydration helps flush bacteria from the urinary tract, reducing the risk of urinary tract infections. UTIs can potentially interfere with fertility.

TO STAY ADEQUATELY HYDRATED, AIM TO:

- Drink plenty of water throughout the day, aiming for at least eight 8-ounce glasses (about 2 liters).
- Pay attention to your body's thirst signals and drink water when you feel thirsty.
- Adjust your fluid intake based on factors like climate, activity level, and individual needs.
- Limit the consumption of dehydrating beverages like caffeine and alcohol.
- Include hydrating foods in your diet, such as fruits and vegetables with high water content.

Remember that hydration is a fundamental aspect of overall health, and maintaining proper hydration is an excellent way to support your fertility journey.

FERTILITY-FRIENDLY DRINK RECIPES.

Here are some fertility-friendly drink recipes that incorporate ingredients known for their potential benefits to reproductive health:

- **FERTILITY-BOOSTING SMOOTHIE:**
- **Ingredients**:
  - 1 cup spinach (rich in folate)
  - 1/2 cup frozen berries (antioxidants)
  - 1 banana (vitamin B6)
  - 1 tablespoon flaxseeds (omega-3 fatty acids)
  - 1/2 cup Greek yogurt (protein)
  - 1/2 cup almond milk (or your preferred milk)
  - 1 teaspoon honey (optional for sweetness)

- **Instructions**:
  1. Blend all ingredients until smooth. Adjust the sweetness with honey, if desired.

- **GINGER-LEMON FERTILITY WATER:**
- **Ingredients**:
  - 1-2 slices of fresh ginger (anti-inflammatory)
  - Juice of 1 lemon (vitamin C)

- 4-6 cups of water

- Optional: a drizzle of honey for sweetness

- **Instructions**:

1. Add ginger slices to a pitcher of water.

2. Squeeze in the lemon juice and add honey if desired.

3. Let it infuse in the refrigerator for a few hours or overnight. Serve chilled.

- **POMEGRANATE BERRY FERTILITY ELIXIR:**

- **Ingredients**:

- 1/2 cup pomegranate juice (rich in antioxidants)
- 1/2 cup mixed berries (vitamin C and antioxidants)
- 1 tablespoon chia seeds (fiber and omega-3s)
- 1 cup coconut water (hydration)

- **Instructions**:

1. Combine pomegranate juice, mixed berries, and chia seeds in a blender.

2. Blend until smooth.

3. Pour into a glass and add coconut water. Stir well and enjoy.

- **CINNAMON AND TURMERIC TEA:**

- **Ingredients**:

- 1 cinnamon stick (anti-inflammatory)

- 1/2 teaspoon ground turmeric (anti-inflammatory)
- 2 cups hot water
- A drizzle of honey (optional)

- **<u>Instructions</u>**:

1. Steep the cinnamon stick and ground turmeric in hot water for 5-10 minutes.

2. Add honey for sweetness, if desired. Sip and enjoy.

- **FERTILITY HERBAL TEA:**

- **<u>Ingredients</u>**:

- 1 teaspoon raspberry leaf (may support uterine health)
- 1 teaspoon nettle leaf (nutrient-rich)
- 1 teaspoon red clover (potential hormonal support)
- 2 cups hot water

- **<u>Instructions</u>**:

1. Steep the herbs in hot water for 5-10 minutes.

2. Strain and enjoy as a caffeine-free herbal tea.

These recipes incorporate fertility-friendly ingredients and can be enjoyed as part of a balanced diet to support your reproductive health. Remember that individual responses to foods and ingredients may vary, so it's always a good idea to consult with a healthcare provider or fertility specialist for personalized guidance.

CAUTION AGAINST EXCESSIVE CAFFEINE AND ALCOHOL.

Excessive caffeine and alcohol consumption can have a negative impact on fertility and reproductive health. Here's why it's essential to exercise caution when it comes to these substances:

- **CAFFEINE:**

1. **Disruption of Hormonal Balance**: Excessive caffeine intake can disrupt hormonal balance, potentially affecting the menstrual cycle in women and sperm quality in men.

2. **Delayed Conception**: Some studies suggest that high caffeine consumption may be associated with longer time to conception.

3. **Increased Miscarriage Risk**: Excessive caffeine intake during pregnancy has been linked to an increased risk of miscarriage. Since many people may not realize they are pregnant in the early stages, it's wise to reduce caffeine intake while actively trying to conceive.

4. **Impact on Ovulation**: In some cases, caffeine may affect ovulation, potentially leading to irregular menstrual cycles.

5. **Stress and Anxiety**: Caffeine is a stimulant that can increase stress and anxiety levels. High stress levels can negatively impact fertility.

6. **Recommendation**: To support fertility, it's advisable for both partners to limit caffeine intake to moderate levels. This typically means consuming no more than 200-400 milligrams (about 1-2 cups of coffee) per day. However, individual sensitivity to caffeine varies, so it's important to listen to your body and adjust accordingly.

- **ALCOHOL:**

1. **Disruption of Hormonal Balance**: Excessive alcohol consumption can interfere with hormonal balance in both men and women, potentially affecting fertility.

2. **Reduced Sperm Quality**: In men, heavy alcohol use has been associated with reduced sperm quality, including decreased sperm count and motility.

3. **Menstrual Irregularities**: In women, excessive alcohol intake can lead to menstrual irregularities, including missed periods.

4. **Increased Risk of Infertility**: Chronic alcohol abuse can lead to liver dysfunction, which may affect hormone metabolism and contribute to infertility.

5. **Impact on Fetal Development**: For women who become pregnant, alcohol consumption during pregnancy can harm fetal development and increase the risk of birth defects.

6. **Recommendation**: To support fertility, it's advisable to limit or avoid alcohol consumption while actively trying to conceive. If you choose to drink alcohol, do so in moderation, and consult with a healthcare provider for personalized guidance.

In summary, it's crucial to exercise caution and moderation when it comes to caffeine and alcohol consumption during the fertility journey. Reducing or eliminating these substances can help optimize reproductive health and increase the chances of a healthy conception and pregnancy. Always consult with a healthcare provider for specific recommendations based on your individual circumstances.

CHAPTER 5:

SPECIAL DIETS AND FERTILITY

In this chapter, we'll explore how various special diets can be adapted to support fertility. Whether you follow a vegetarian, vegan, gluten-free, or other specific dietary plan, you can make choices that align with your dietary preferences while also enhancing your reproductive health.

• VEGETARIAN DIETS AND FERTILITY

- **Balancing Nutrients**: Tips for ensuring you get enough protein, iron, and vitamin B12 from plant-based sources.

- **Plant-Based Protein Sources**: A list of protein-rich foods suitable for vegetarians to support fertility.

-**Fertility-Friendly Vegetarian Recipes**: Delicious plant-based recipes tailored for reproductive health.

• VEGAN DIETS AND FERTILITY

- **Meeting Nutritional Needs:** Guidance on obtaining essential nutrients like vitamin B12, iron, calcium, and omega-3 fatty acids on a vegan diet.

- **Plant-Based Omega-3 Sources:** Explore vegan sources of omega-3s that benefit reproductive health.

- **Vegan-Friendly Fertility Recipes:** Nutrient-dense vegan recipes designed to support fertility.

- **GLUTEN-FREE DIETS AND FERTILITY**
- **Understanding Celiac Disease**: How celiac disease can impact fertility and strategies for managing it.
- **Navigating Gluten-Free Grains**: Identifying gluten-free grains like quinoa and rice that can be part of a fertility-focused diet.
- **Gluten-Free Fertility Meal Plans:** Sample meal plans for individuals with celiac disease or gluten sensitivity.

- **LOW-CARB DIETS AND FERTILITY**
-**Balancing Carbohydrates**: Exploring how low-carb diets can be adjusted to include fertility-friendly carbohydrates.
-**Healthy Fats and Proteins**: Emphasizing sources of healthy fats and proteins to support reproductive health.
-**Low-Carb Fertility-Focused Recipes**: Recipes that align with low-carb dietary preferences while boosting fertility.

- **FOOD ALLERGIES AND FERTILITY**
-**Managing Food Allergies:** Strategies for individuals with food allergies, including dairy, nuts, or eggs, while maintaining a fertility-conscious diet.
-**Substitutes and Alternatives**: Identifying suitable substitutes for allergenic foods in fertility-friendly recipes.

-**Allergy-Friendly Fertility Recipes:** Recipes tailored for individuals with common food allergies.

- **HOLISTIC APPROACHES TO SPECIAL DIETS**

-**Consulting with a Dietitian:** The importance of seeking guidance from a registered dietitian or healthcare professional when following a special diet for fertility.

-**Supplements and Specialized Diets**: Exploring the role of supplements and specialized dietary plans in fertility, such as the Mediterranean diet or the ketogenic diet.

By the end of this chapter, you'll have a comprehensive understanding of how to adapt special diets to support fertility. Whether you have specific dietary restrictions or preferences, you can make choices that align with your needs while nurturing your reproductive health on your journey to parenthood.

VEGAN AND VEGETARIAN OPTIONS

For individuals following vegan and vegetarian diets, it's essential to make mindful food choices to ensure you're getting the necessary nutrients to support fertility. Here are some vegan and vegetarian options tailored for reproductive health:

- **VEGAN AND VEGETARIAN PROTEIN SOURCES:**

Vegan Options: Incorporate plant-based proteins like tofu, tempeh, legumes (lentils, chickpeas, black beans), and edamame.

Vegetarian Options: Include dairy products (Greek yogurt, cottage cheese) and eggs as additional protein sources.

- **PLANT-BASED OMEGA-3 FATS:**

Vegan Options: Chia seeds, flaxseeds, hemp seeds, and walnuts are rich in alpha-linolenic acid (ALA), a type of omega-3 fatty acid.

Vegetarian Options: Fatty fish like salmon and trout are excellent sources of omega-3s. Consider incorporating these if you're a vegetarian.

- **FOLATE-RICH FOODS:**

__Vegan Options__: Dark leafy greens (spinach, kale), asparagus, and broccoli are folate-rich vegetables.

__Vegetarian Options__: Eggs and dairy products like yogurt and cheese are good sources of folate for vegetarians.

- **IRON-RICH PLANT FOODS:**

__Vegan Options__: Incorporate iron-rich foods like lentils, fortified cereals, and spinach. Pair them with vitamin C-rich foods to enhance iron absorption.

__Vegetarian Options:__ Eggs and dairy products also provide iron for vegetarians.

- **CALCIUM SOURCES:**

__Vegan Options__: Fortified plant-based milk (almond milk, soy milk), tofu, and leafy greens (collard greens, bok choy) are sources of calcium.

__Vegetarian Options:__ Dairy products like yogurt and cheese are excellent sources of calcium for vegetarians.

- **B12 SUPPLEMENTATION:**

Vitamin B12 is primarily found in animal products, so it's essential for vegans to take B12 supplements or consume B12-fortified foods like plant-based milk or cereals.

- **PLANT-BASED FIBER:**

Fiber is important for digestive health. Whole grains like quinoa, brown rice, and oats, as well as fruits and vegetables, provide essential fiber for vegans and vegetarians.

- **HYDRATION:**

Staying well-hydrated is vital for reproductive health for both vegans and vegetarians. Drink plenty of water throughout the day.

- **BALANCED MEALS:**

Ensure your meals are balanced with a variety of vegetables, whole grains, and plant-based proteins to provide essential nutrients for fertility.

- **CONSULT A DIETITIAN:**

For personalized guidance, consider consulting a registered dietitian who specializes in plant-based nutrition to ensure you're meeting your nutritional needs for fertility.

Adapting a vegan or vegetarian diet to support fertility is entirely feasible with proper planning and food choices. By incorporating these options and consulting with a dietitian when needed, you can nurture your reproductive health while following your preferred dietary lifestyle.

GLUTEN-FREE AND FERTILITY

Individuals who follow a gluten-free diet, either due to celiac disease or non-celiac gluten sensitivity, can still support their fertility with a well-balanced and nutritious eating plan. Here are considerations for those on a gluten-free diet:

- **GLUTEN-FREE WHOLE GRAINS:**

  - Incorporate gluten-free whole grains like quinoa, brown rice, millet, and certified gluten-free oats into your diet. These provide essential carbohydrates and fiber.

  - Avoid gluten-containing grains like wheat, barley, and rye, which can trigger adverse reactions if you have celiac disease or gluten sensitivity.

- **FOLATE-RICH FOODS:**

  - Consume folate-rich foods such as leafy greens, legumes (lentils, chickpeas), and fortified gluten-free cereals.

  - Check food labels to ensure gluten-free products are fortified with essential nutrients like folate.

- **LEAN PROTEINS:**

- Include lean protein sources like poultry, fish, tofu, tempeh, beans, and nuts in your gluten-free meals. These support reproductive health.

- Avoid breaded or battered proteins, as they often contain gluten.

- **DAIRY OR DAIRY ALTERNATIVES:**

- Dairy products and dairy alternatives like almond milk, soy milk, or lactose-free options can provide calcium and vitamin D.

- Check labels to confirm they are gluten-free.

- **GLUTEN-FREE FIBER:**

- Choose gluten-free fiber sources such as fruits, vegetables, gluten-free whole grains, and gluten-free oats.

- Fiber supports digestive health and hormonal balance.

- **GLUTEN-FREE SNACKS:**

- Opt for gluten-free snacks like nuts, seeds, gluten-free rice cakes, and vegetable sticks with gluten-free hummus.

- Avoid processed snacks that may contain gluten.

- **GLUTEN-FREE SUPPLEMENTS:**

- If you have celiac disease, consult with a healthcare professional to determine if you need gluten-free supplements for specific nutrients.

- Some supplements may contain gluten as a binding agent.

- **GLUTEN-FREE LABEL READING:**

- Familiarize yourself with gluten-free labeling and certifications to ensure the safety of your food choices.

- Be cautious when dining out and inquire about gluten-free options and food preparation practices.

- **HYDRATION:**

- Stay well-hydrated with water and gluten-free beverages to support overall health and reproductive wellness.

For individuals with celiac disease, strictly adhering to a gluten-free diet is critical to prevent intestinal damage and promote optimal nutrient absorption. If you have concerns or questions about how a gluten-free diet may impact your fertility, consider consulting with a registered dietitian or healthcare professional experienced in gluten-free nutrition for personalized guidance.

ALLERGIES AND FERTILITY
Navigating Food Allergies on Your Fertility Journey

Managing food allergies while trying to conceive or during pregnancy requires careful attention to ensure both the safety of the individual with allergies and the nourishment needed for fertility and a healthy pregnancy. Here's how to navigate common food allergies and their impact on fertility:

- **DAIRY ALLERGIES:**
- **Alternatives**: If you have a dairy allergy, consider lactose-free or plant-based milk alternatives like almond, soy, or oat milk.

  -**Calcium Intake:** Ensure you're getting enough calcium from fortified dairy-free products or supplements.

- **NUT ALLERGIES:**
-**Nut-Free Proteins:** Opt for protein sources that don't involve nuts, such as lean meats, poultry, fish, beans, and legumes.

  - **Read Labels**: Be vigilant about reading food labels to avoid products that may contain hidden nuts.

- **EGG ALLERGIES:**

- **Substitutes**: In recipes that call for eggs, use egg substitutes like applesauce, mashed bananas, or commercial egg replacers.

- **Protein Sources**: Seek protein from sources like lean meats, poultry, fish, tofu, or legumes.

- **SHELLFISH AND SEAFOOD ALLERGIES:**

- **Alternatives**: If you have seafood allergies, ensure you're obtaining essential omega-3 fatty acids from plant-based sources like flaxseed, chia seeds, or algae-based supplements.

- **Diverse Protein Choices**: Explore a variety of protein options beyond seafood, such as poultry, lean meats, tofu, or beans.

- **WHEAT AND GLUTEN ALLERGIES:**

-**Gluten-Free Grains**: Embrace gluten-free whole grains like quinoa, brown rice, millet, and certified gluten-free oats for carbohydrates.

- **Folate Sources:** Focus on folate-rich foods like leafy greens, lentils, and chickpeas to compensate for the absence of wheat products.

- **ALLERGEN-FREE SUPPLEMENTS:**

- When dietary restrictions limit your nutrient intake, consider allergen-free supplements or prenatal vitamins that accommodate your specific allergies.

- Consult a healthcare professional for guidance on suitable supplements.

• BALANCED MEALS:

- Ensure your meals are well-balanced, incorporating a variety of allergen-free foods to support fertility and overall health.

- Work with a registered dietitian to create meal plans tailored to your dietary needs.

• CONSULTATION WITH AN ALLERGIST:

- If you have severe food allergies, consult with an allergist to manage your allergies effectively and minimize risks.

Managing food allergies and maintaining a fertility-conscious diet is entirely achievable with proper planning, ingredient substitutions, and awareness of allergen-containing products. Prioritize open communication with healthcare providers, including allergists and dietitians, to ensure your dietary choices align with your fertility goals and overall well-being.

CHAPTER 6:

SUPERFOODS FOR FERTILITY

Superfoods are nutrient-dense, powerhouse ingredients that can provide a significant boost to reproductive health. In this chapter, we'll explore a variety of superfoods that can enhance fertility for both partners:

- **BERRIES FOR ANTIOXIDANT POWER**

- Learn how berries like blueberries, strawberries, and raspberries can improve fertility through their high antioxidant content.

- Discover creative ways to incorporate berries into your diet, from smoothie bowls to yogurt parfaits.

- **LEAFY GREENS FOR FOLATE AND NUTRIENTS**

- Understand the importance of folate-rich leafy greens like spinach, kale, and collard greens for healthy egg development and overall fertility.

- Explore recipes that make these greens a delicious addition to your meals.

- **FATTY FISH FOR OMEGA-3S**

- Explore the benefits of fatty fish like salmon, mackerel, and sardines in regulating hormones and supporting reproductive health.

- Learn how to prepare and include these fish in your diet for maximum fertility benefits.

- **AVOCADO FOR HEALTHY FATS**

- Discover how avocados' healthy fats can help regulate hormones and improve fertility.

- Explore recipes that incorporate avocados, from smoothies to salads.

- **NUTS AND SEEDS FOR NUTRIENT DENSITY**

- Learn about the nutrient-rich qualities of nuts and seeds like almonds, walnuts, chia seeds, and flaxseeds.

- Find out how to integrate these superfoods into your daily meals and snacks.

- **BEANS AND LENTILS FOR PLANT-BASED PROTEIN**

- Explore the fertility benefits of beans and lentils, which provide plant-based protein, fiber, and essential nutrients.

- Discover recipes that showcase these legumes in flavorful and nourishing ways.

- **OYSTERS AND ZINC**

- Understand the role of zinc in fertility and how oysters are an excellent source of this essential mineral.

- Explore ways to incorporate zinc-rich foods into your diet.

- **DARK CHOCOLATE FOR ANTIOXIDANTS**
- Learn how dark chocolate with a high cocoa content can provide antioxidants that support reproductive health.
- Enjoy guilt-free dark chocolate recipes that cater to your sweet cravings.

- **POMEGRANATES FOR FERTILITY BOOST**
- Discover the potential fertility-boosting properties of pomegranates and their antioxidants.
- Explore creative ways to enjoy pomegranates, from juices to salad toppings.

- **HERBAL TEAS FOR RELAXATION AND HYDRATION**
- Explore herbal teas like chamomile and peppermint, which can aid in relaxation and hydration during your fertility journey.

- **INTEGRATING SUPERFOODS INTO MEAL PLANS**

- Learn how to create balanced meal plans that incorporate these superfoods, ensuring you reap their fertility benefits.
- Get inspired with sample meal plans and recipes designed around these nutrient-rich ingredients.

By the end of this chapter, you'll have a comprehensive understanding of how superfoods can play a vital role in enhancing your fertility. You'll also have a variety of delicious recipes and meal plans to help you integrate these superfoods into your daily diet, setting you on a path to improved reproductive health.

THE POWER OF ANTIOXIDANTS

Antioxidants are crucial compounds that can positively impact fertility for both partners. They help protect reproductive cells from oxidative stress, which can damage sperm, eggs, and reproductive organs. Here's why antioxidants are a vital component of a fertility-focused diet:

- **REDUCING OXIDATIVE STRESS:**
  - Oxidative stress occurs when there's an imbalance between free radicals (harmful molecules) and antioxidants in the body.
  - High levels of oxidative stress can harm sperm DNA, impair egg quality, and disrupt hormone balance.

- **SPERM HEALTH:**
  - Antioxidants like vitamin C, vitamin E, and selenium can improve sperm quality by reducing DNA damage and enhancing sperm motility.
  - Adequate antioxidant intake can increase the chances of successful fertilization.

- **EGG QUALITY:**
  - Antioxidants can help protect eggs from oxidative damage, potentially leading to healthier embryos.
  - This is particularly important for women, as egg quality plays a crucial role in conception and healthy pregnancy.

- **HORMONAL BALANCE:**

- Antioxidants support hormonal balance by neutralizing harmful compounds that can disrupt the endocrine system.

- Balanced hormones are essential for regular menstrual cycles and ovulation.

- **INFLAMMATION REDUCTION:**

- Chronic inflammation can negatively impact fertility. Antioxidants combat inflammation, creating a more conducive environment for conception.

- **REPRODUCTIVE ORGAN HEALTH:**

- Antioxidants contribute to the overall health of the reproductive organs, including the uterus and fallopian tubes.

- A healthy reproductive system is more likely to support conception and a successful pregnancy.

- **FERTILITY SUPERFOODS:**

- Many superfoods, such as berries, dark chocolate, and pomegranates, are rich in antioxidants and can be incorporated into a fertility-focused diet.

- **SUPPLEMENTATION:**

- In some cases, couples may benefit from antioxidant supplements. Consult a healthcare provider or fertility specialist for personalized recommendations.

- **DIET AND LIFESTYLE:**

- Maintaining a diet rich in fruits, vegetables, whole grains, and nuts is a natural way to increase antioxidant intake.

- Lifestyle factors like regular exercise and stress reduction also contribute to overall antioxidant support.

- **TIMING MATTERS:**

- Consuming antioxidant-rich foods regularly, rather than sporadically, can help maintain a consistent level of protection against oxidative stress.

By including antioxidant-rich foods in your diet and adopting a lifestyle that reduces oxidative stress, you can harness the power of antioxidants to enhance your fertility journey. Remember that a balanced and nutrient-rich diet, along with other healthy habits, can make a significant difference in your reproductive health.

OMEGA-3 FATTY ACIDS AND FERTILITY

Omega-3 fatty acids are a group of essential fats that offer a range of health benefits, including support for fertility and reproductive health. Here's how omega-3s can positively impact your fertility journey:

- **REGULATION OF HORMONES:**

- Omega-3s help regulate hormone production and function, which is essential for both men and women trying to conceive.

- Hormone balance is crucial for ovulation in women and sperm production in men.

- **IMPROVING EGG QUALITY:**

- For women, omega-3 fatty acids can enhance egg quality by reducing inflammation and oxidative stress.

- Better egg quality increases the likelihood of successful conception.

- **ENHANCING SPERM QUALITY:**

- In men, omega-3s can improve sperm quality by enhancing motility and reducing DNA damage.

- High-quality sperm are vital for fertilization and a healthy pregnancy.

- **REDUCING INFLAMMATION:**
- Omega-3s have anti-inflammatory properties that can help individuals with conditions like endometriosis or polycystic ovary syndrome (PCOS).
- Lowering inflammation can improve overall reproductive health.

- **SUPPORTING THE MENSTRUAL CYCLE:**
- Omega-3s can help regulate the menstrual cycle, making it more predictable and consistent.
- Regular menstrual cycles are important for timing ovulation and conception.

- **BLOOD FLOW IMPROVEMENT:**
- Some omega-3s, particularly those found in fatty fish like salmon and mackerel, can improve blood flow to reproductive organs.
- Enhanced blood circulation ensures these organs receive the necessary nutrients.

- **OMEGA-3-RICH FOODS:**
- Fatty fish (salmon, mackerel, sardines)
- Chia seeds
- Flaxseeds
- Walnuts
- Hemp seeds
- Algal oil (a plant-based source of omega-3s for vegans)

- Fish oil supplements (consult a healthcare provider before taking supplements)

Incorporating omega-3-rich foods into your diet or considering supplements can be a valuable addition to your fertility-focused nutrition plan. However, it's essential to maintain a balanced diet that includes various nutrients for overall reproductive health. If you have specific concerns about fertility or dietary needs, consult with a healthcare professional or registered dietitian for personalized guidance.

HERBS AND SUPPLEMENTS

While a balanced diet is essential for fertility, some herbs and supplements may complement your nutrition and support reproductive health. Here are some commonly considered options:

- **FOLATE OR FOLIC ACID:**
  - Essential for healthy pregnancy and fetal development.
  - Often included in prenatal vitamins, but it's advisable to consult a healthcare provider for the appropriate dosage.

- **COENZYME Q10 (COQ10):**
  - An antioxidant that may improve egg and sperm quality.
  - Consult a healthcare provider for the correct dosage.

- **VITEX (CHASTE TREE BERRY):**
  - May help regulate the menstrual cycle and hormonal balance in women.
  - Consult with a healthcare provider before use, especially if you have hormonal disorders or are taking medications.

- **IRON SUPPLEMENTS:**
  - Important for women with iron-deficiency anemia, which can affect fertility.

- Consult a healthcare provider for personalized recommendations.

- **VITAMIN D:**
- Plays a role in hormone regulation and reproductive health.
- Consult with a healthcare provider to determine if supplementation is necessary.

- **OMEGA-3 FATTY ACID SUPPLEMENTS:**
- Especially beneficial if you have difficulty incorporating omega-3-rich foods into your diet.
- Consult with a healthcare provider for the correct dosage.

- **ACETYL-L-CARNITINE AND L-CARNITINE:**
- May improve sperm quality and motility in men.
- Consult with a healthcare provider before use.

- **HERBAL TEAS:**
- Some herbal teas, like red raspberry leaf tea, may support uterine health and menstrual regularity.
- Consult with a healthcare provider or herbalist for guidance.

- **MACA ROOT:**

- Believed to enhance fertility and libido, particularly in men.

- Consult with a healthcare provider before use, especially if you have hormonal disorders.

- **PRECONCEPTION AND PRENATAL VITAMINS:**
  - These often contain a combination of essential vitamins and minerals for reproductive health.
  - Consult with a healthcare provider to choose the right supplement for your needs.

- **ZINC SUPPLEMENTS:**
  - Important for sperm production and motility in men.
  - Consult with a healthcare provider for personalized recommendations.

- **HERBAL SUPPLEMENTS FOR MENSTRUAL HEALTH:**
  - Supplements like evening primrose oil or chasteberry may be considered to regulate the menstrual cycle in women.
  - Consult with a healthcare provider or herbalist for guidance.

- **IMPORTANT NOTES:**

- Always consult with a healthcare provider, especially a reproductive endocrinologist or a fertility specialist, before starting any new supplements or herbs.
- Individual needs vary, and what works for one person may not work for another.
- Supplements should complement a well-balanced diet and not replace it.

Remember that supplements should be used under the guidance of a healthcare professional, as taking excessive or unnecessary supplements can have adverse effects on health. A healthcare provider can help assess your specific fertility needs and recommend the appropriate supplements or herbs tailored to your situation.

CHAPTER 7:

MEAL PLANS AND RECIPES

In this chapter, we'll provide you with comprehensive meal plans and delicious recipes designed to nourish your reproductive health. Whether you're trying to conceive or simply aiming to support your fertility journey, these meal plans and recipes will help you maintain a balanced and nutritious diet.

ONE-WEEK MEAL PLAN FOR HER

Here is a one-week meal plan designed to support women's fertility. This plan includes a variety of nutrient-rich foods and fertility-boosting ingredients.

- **DAY 1:**

Breakfast:
Greek yogurt parfait with berries and almonds
Lunch:
Quinoa and chickpea salad with mixed greens
Snack:
Carrot and cucumber sticks with hummus
Dinner:
Grilled salmon with asparagus and quinoa

- **DAY 2:**

Breakfast: Spinach and mushroom omelette with a side of whole-grain toast

<u>Lunch</u>:

Lentil soup with a side of mixed greens

<u>Snack</u>:

Greek yogurt with honey and walnuts

<u>Dinner</u>:

Vegetable stir-fry with tofu and brown rice

- **DAY 3:**

<u>Breakfast:</u>

Smoothie with spinach, banana, chia seeds, and almond milk

<u>Lunch:</u>

Avocado and black bean salad with a lime-cilantro dressing

<u>Snack:</u>

Mixed berries and a handful of almonds

<u>Dinner</u>:

Baked sweet potato with black bean chili

- **DAY 4:**

<u>Breakfast</u>:

Overnight oats with sliced strawberries and flaxseeds

<u>Lunch</u>:

Whole-grain pasta with tomato and vegetable sauce

<u>Snack</u>:

Sliced cucumber and cherry tomatoes with balsamic vinaigrette

Dinner:

Grilled chicken breast with quinoa and roasted broccoli

- **DAY 5:**

Breakfast:

Cottage cheese with sliced peaches and a sprinkle of sunflower seeds

Lunch:

Spinach and feta stuffed bell peppers

Snack:

Apple slices with almond butter

Dinner:

Homemade sushi rolls with avocado, cucumber, and salmon

- **DAY 6:**

Breakfast:

Whole-grain waffles with Greek yogurt and fresh berries

Lunch:

Quinoa salad with roasted vegetables and feta cheese

Snack: Edamame with a sprinkle of sea salt

Dinner: Portobello mushroom burgers with a side salad

- **DAY 7:**

Breakfast:

Scrambled eggs with spinach and tomatoes

<u>Lunch:</u>
Lentil and vegetable curry with brown rice
<u>Snack</u>:
Sliced bell peppers with hummus
<u>Dinner:</u>
Grilled vegetable and chickpea salad with a lemon-tahini dressing

Remember to drink plenty of water throughout the day to stay hydrated. This meal plan incorporates a variety of fertility-friendly foods, including leafy greens, berries, whole grains, lean proteins, and healthy fats. It's essential to maintain a balanced diet to support reproductive health. Feel free to adapt these meals to your preferences and dietary requirements.

ONE-WEEK MEAL PLAN FOR HIM
And here is a one-week meal plan designed to support men's fertility. This plan includes a variety of nutrient-rich foods and fertility-boosting ingredients.

- **DAY 1:**

Breakfast:
Scrambled eggs with spinach and whole-grain toast
Lunch:
Turkey and avocado wrap with mixed greens
Snack:
Greek yogurt with honey and almonds
Dinner:
Grilled chicken breast with quinoa and steamed broccoli

- **DAY 2:**

Breakfast:
Oatmeal with sliced bananas and walnuts
Lunch:
Lentil soup with a side of mixed greens
Snack:
Sliced cucumber and carrot sticks with hummus
Dinner:
Baked salmon with quinoa and roasted Brussels sprouts

- **DAY 3:**

Breakfast:

Smoothie with kale, banana, chia seeds, and almond milk

Lunch:

Quinoa salad with chickpeas, tomatoes, and feta cheese

Snack:

Mixed berries and a handful of pistachios

Dinner:

Grilled steak with sweet potato and grilled asparagus

- **DAY 4:**

Breakfast:

Greek yogurt parfait with berries and flax seeds

Lunch:

Turkey and black bean salad with a balsamic vinaigrette

Snack:

Apple slices with almond butter

Dinner:

Grilled shrimp with brown rice and sautéed spinach

- **DAY 5:**

Breakfast:

Scrambled eggs with diced tomatoes and whole-grain toast

Lunch:

Quinoa and vegetable stir-fry with tofu

<u>**Snack**</u>:

Sliced bell peppers and cherry tomatoes with ranch dressing

<u>**Dinner:**</u>

Beef and vegetable kebabs with a side of quinoa

- **DAY 6:**

<u>**Breakfast:**</u>

Whole-grain waffles with Greek yogurt and fresh strawberries

<u>**Lunch:**</u>

Spinach and mushroom omelette with a side of mixed greens

<u>**Snack**</u>:

Edamame with a sprinkle of sea salt

<u>**Dinner:**</u>

Baked chicken thighs with brown rice and steamed broccoli

- **DAY 7:**

<u>**Breakfast:**</u>

Cottage cheese with pineapple chunks and a sprinkle of sunflower seeds

<u>**Lunch**</u>:

Turkey chili with a side of whole-grain crackers

<u>**Snack**</u>:

Mixed nuts and dried fruit

<u>Dinner</u>:

Grilled pork chops with sweet potato fries and sautéed green beans

Staying well-hydrated throughout the day is essential, so be sure to drink plenty of water. This meal plan includes a variety of fertility-friendly foods, including lean proteins, whole grains, fruits, vegetables, and healthy fats. Feel free to adjust these meals to your preferences and dietary requirements. Supporting overall health and fertility with a balanced diet is key for both partners on the fertility journey.

DELICIOUS FERTILITY-FOCUSED RECIPES

Below are some delicious fertility-focused recipes for both partners on your fertility journey:

FERTILITY-BOOSTING SMOOTHIE BOWL:
- **<u>Ingredients</u>**:
    - 1 cup mixed berries (blueberries, strawberries, raspberries)
    - 1 banana
    - 1/2 cup Greek yogurt
    - 1 tablespoon chia seeds
    - 1 tablespoon honey
    - 1/4 cup granola

- **<u>Instructions</u>**:
    1. Blend the mixed berries, banana, Greek yogurt, chia seeds, and honey until smooth.
    2. Pour the smoothie into a bowl.
    3. Top with granola, more berries, and a drizzle of honey.

QUINOA AND CHICKPEA SALAD:
- **<u>Ingredients</u>**:
    - 1 cup cooked quinoa
    - 1 can chickpeas, drained and rinsed
    - 1 cup diced cucumber
    - 1 cup cherry tomatoes, halved
    - 1/4 cup chopped fresh parsley

- 2 tablespoons olive oil
- Juice of 1 lemon
- Salt and pepper to taste

- **<u>Instructions</u>**:

1. In a large bowl, combine the quinoa, chickpeas, cucumber, cherry tomatoes, and parsley.

2. In a small bowl, whisk together the olive oil and lemon juice. Season with salt and pepper.

3. Pour the dressing over the salad and toss to combine. Serve chilled.

GRILLED SALMON WITH ASPARAGUS AND QUINOA:

- **<u>Ingredients</u>**:
  - 2 salmon fillets
  - 1 bunch asparagus, trimmed
  - 1 cup cooked quinoa
  - Zest and juice of 1 lemon
  - 2 cloves garlic, minced
  - 2 tablespoons olive oil
  - Salt and pepper to taste

- **<u>Instructions</u>**:

1. Preheat the grill to medium-high heat.

2. In a small bowl, whisk together the lemon zest, lemon juice, minced garlic, olive oil, salt, and pepper.

3. Brush the salmon and asparagus with the lemon-garlic mixture.

4. Grill the salmon for about 4-5 minutes per side and the asparagus for 2-3 minutes, until tender.

5. Serve the grilled salmon and asparagus over a bed of cooked quinoa.

SPINACH AND MUSHROOM OMELETTE:

- **<u>Ingredients</u>**:
  - 3 large eggs
  - 1 cup fresh spinach leaves
  - 1/2 cup sliced mushrooms
  - 1/4 cup diced tomatoes
  - 2 tablespoons shredded cheese (optional)
  - Salt and pepper to taste

- **<u>Instructions</u>**:
  1. In a bowl, beat the eggs and season with salt and pepper.
  2. Heat a non-stick skillet over medium heat and lightly coat it with cooking spray.
  3. Add the mushrooms and cook for 2-3 minutes until they start to brown.
  4. Add the spinach and tomatoes to the skillet and sauté until the spinach wilts.
  5. Pour the beaten eggs over the vegetables and cook until the edges start to set.
  6. Sprinkle shredded cheese on top if desired.

7. Fold the omelette in half and cook for another 1-2 minutes until it's fully set. Serve hot.

These recipes are not only delicious but also packed with fertility-friendly ingredients to support your reproductive health. Enjoy these meals as part of your balanced diet on your fertility journey.

CHAPTER 8:

DINING OUT AND SOCIAL SITUATIONS

Maintaining a fertility-focused diet doesn't mean you have to avoid dining out or social gatherings. In this chapter, we'll explore strategies and tips for navigating various dining scenarios while staying true to your fertility goals. You'll learn how to make informed choices at restaurants, attend parties, and handle social situations with ease.

NAVIGATING RESTAURANTS

Dining out at restaurants can be enjoyable without compromising your fertility-focused nutrition. Here are some strategies to help you make informed choices when dining at restaurants:

- **Review the Menu in Advance:**
  - Many restaurants now have their menus available online. Take a look before you go to identify fertility-friendly options.

- **Choose Lean Proteins:**
  - Opt for dishes that feature lean proteins like grilled chicken, turkey, fish, or tofu. These provide essential nutrients without excess saturated fat.

- **Load Up on Veggies:**

- Incorporate vegetables into your meal by choosing dishes with generous vegetable servings or ordering a side salad or steamed vegetables.

- **Go for Whole Grains:**

- Select dishes with whole grains such as brown rice, quinoa, or whole wheat pasta. These grains are rich in fiber and nutrients.

- **Be Mindful of Portion Sizes:**

- Pay attention to portion sizes, as restaurant servings are often larger than necessary. Consider sharing an entrée or taking leftovers home.

- **Ask for Modifications:**

- Don't hesitate to ask the server for modifications to your dish. For example, request that your meal be prepared with less oil or butter.

- **Watch Sauces and Dressings:**

- Be cautious of heavy sauces and dressings, which can be high in calories and saturated fats. Ask for sauces on the side or choose dishes with lighter sauces.

- **Limit Alcohol and Sugary Drinks:**

- Opt for water, herbal tea, or sparkling water instead of sugary beverages or excessive alcohol. Alcohol can affect fertility, so consume it in moderation.

- **Avoid Deep-Fried Foods:**

- Steer clear of deep-fried foods, as they are often high in unhealthy fats and can contribute to inflammation.

- **Mindful Eating:**

- Practice mindful eating by savoring each bite and paying attention to your body's hunger and fullness cues.

- **Dessert Alternatives:**

- Instead of rich desserts, consider ordering fresh fruit or sharing a dessert with your dining companion.

- **Be Assertive but Polite:**

- Don't hesitate to communicate your dietary preferences to the server politely. Most restaurants are accommodating.

Remember that dining out should be an enjoyable experience. You can make choices that align with your fertility-focused diet while still savoring delicious restaurant meals. It's about balance and making informed decisions that support your goals.

FERTILITY-FRIENDLY CHOICES AT SOCIAL GATHERINGS

Maintaining a fertility-focused diet at social gatherings is possible with some thoughtful choices. Here are tips for navigating various social situations while staying true to your fertility goals:

- **Plan Ahead:**
- If possible, find out in advance what food will be served at the gathering. This can help you prepare mentally and make informed choices.

- **Bring a Dish:**
- Offer to bring a fertility-friendly dish to share. This ensures you have a nutritious option and introduces others to healthy choices.

- **Focus on Veggies:**
- Load your plate with vegetables if they're available. Opt for salads, vegetable platters, or roasted vegetables.

- **Lean Proteins:**
- Choose protein sources like grilled chicken, fish, or tofu if they are offered. They're usually healthier than heavily processed meats.

- **Control Portions:**

- Be mindful of portion sizes. Take a small portion of indulgent dishes and fill the rest of your plate with healthier options.

- **Watch Sugary Drinks:**

- Be cautious with sugary cocktails and soft drinks. Opt for sparkling water with a splash of citrus or herbal tea.

- **Limit Alcohol:**

- If you consume alcohol, do so in moderation. Excessive alcohol intake can negatively impact fertility.

- **Practice Moderation:**

- It's okay to indulge occasionally, but practice moderation. Enjoy a small piece of cake or a scoop of ice cream without guilt.

- **Stay Hydrated**:

- Drink plenty of water throughout the event to stay hydrated.

- **Be Selective with Desserts:**

- If dessert is a must, choose options with fresh fruit or lower sugar content. Alternatively, share a dessert with someone.

- **Socialize Away from the Buffet:**

- Engage in conversations away from the food table to minimize mindless snacking.

- **Communicate Your Goals:**

- If you're comfortable, let your close friends or family know about your fertility goals. They can provide support and understanding.

- **Enjoy the Company:**

- Remember that social gatherings are not just about the food. Focus on enjoying the company of friends and loved ones.

- **Be Kind to Yourself:**

- If you do indulge more than planned, don't be too hard on yourself. One day of indulgence won't derail your fertility journey.

Balancing social gatherings with your fertility goals is about making thoughtful choices while still savoring the moments with friends and family. It's possible to enjoy these events while maintaining a fertility-conscious approach to your diet.

CHAPTER 9:

LIFESTYLE AND FERTILITY

Your lifestyle plays a crucial role in your fertility journey. In this chapter, we'll explore the various lifestyle factors that can impact reproductive health. You'll learn how to make positive lifestyle changes that can enhance your chances of conceiving and promote a healthy pregnancy.

- **Stress Management and Fertility**
- Strategies for managing stress and its impact on fertility.
- Techniques such as meditation, yoga, and mindfulness to reduce stress.

- **Exercise and Fertility**
- The relationship between physical activity and reproductive health.
- Guidance on the right balance of exercise for fertility.

- **Sleep and Reproductive Health**
- The importance of sleep in maintaining hormonal balance and fertility.
- Tips for improving sleep quality and duration.

- **Smoking, Alcohol, and Fertility**
- The effects of smoking and excessive alcohol consumption on fertility.

- Strategies for quitting smoking and moderating alcohol intake.

- **Weight and Fertility**
- How body weight and fertility are interconnected.
- Guidance on achieving and maintaining a healthy weight for fertility.

- **Environmental Toxins and Fertility**
- Understanding the impact of environmental toxins on reproductive health.
- Tips for reducing exposure to harmful chemicals.

- **Relationships and Support**
- The importance of a supportive partner and network during the fertility journey.
- Strategies for open communication and emotional support.

- **Mind-Body Connection and Fertility**
- The connection between mental well-being and reproductive health.
- Techniques for fostering a positive mindset and emotional balance.

- **Preconception Care and Healthcare Providers**
- The role of preconception care in optimizing fertility.

- How to choose a healthcare provider and the importance of regular check-ups.

By the end of this chapter, you'll have a comprehensive understanding of how lifestyle choices and practices can impact fertility. You'll also gain practical insights into making positive changes that support your reproductive health and increase your chances of conceiving.

EXERCISE AND FERTILITY

Exercise can have a significant impact on fertility, but finding the right balance is key. Here's how exercise can affect your fertility journey and some guidelines to help you strike the right balance:

- **Benefits of Exercise for Fertility:**
- Regular, moderate exercise can improve overall health, which is essential for fertility.
- It helps maintain a healthy body weight, which can enhance reproductive function.
- Exercise can reduce stress, which may positively influence fertility.
- It can help regulate menstrual cycles and ovulation in some women.

- **Moderation is Key:**
- Excessive exercise, such as intense training for marathons or triathlons, can disrupt menstrual cycles and ovulation.
- Overexercising may lead to low body fat levels, which can affect hormonal balance and fertility.
- Striking a balance between staying active and avoiding excessive exercise is crucial.

- **Recommended Exercise Guidelines:**
- Aim for at least 150 minutes of moderate-intensity exercise per week, or 75 minutes of vigorous-intensity exercise, according to the American College of Obstetricians and Gynecologists (ACOG).
- Incorporate a mix of aerobic activities (e.g., walking, jogging, cycling) and strength training exercises.
- Listen to your body. If you experience irregular periods, missed periods, or other menstrual irregularities, consider reducing the intensity or duration of your workouts.

- **Avoid Extreme Dieting:**
- Coupling intense exercise with extreme calorie restriction can negatively affect fertility.
- Ensure that you're eating enough to support your energy expenditure, especially if you engage in regular workouts.

- **Consult a Healthcare Provider:**
- If you're concerned about the impact of exercise on your fertility, consult a healthcare provider or fertility specialist.
- They can assess your individual situation and provide guidance tailored to your needs.

- **Focus on Stress Reduction:**

- While moderate exercise can reduce stress, excessive exercise may have the opposite effect.

- Consider incorporating stress-reduction practices like yoga or meditation into your routine.

- **Partner Communication:**

- If you're trying to conceive as a couple, ensure open communication with your partner about exercise habits and goals.

- **Preconception Care:**

- If you plan to conceive, consider preconception care, which involves optimizing your health before pregnancy. This may include adjusting exercise and nutrition habits.

Remember that the impact of exercise on fertility can vary from person to person. The key is to find a healthy balance that supports your overall well-being while promoting reproductive health. If you have concerns or specific questions about exercise and fertility, consult with a healthcare provider or reproductive specialist for personalized guidance.

STRESS MANAGEMENT AND FERTILITY

Stress can have a significant impact on fertility for both men and women. Here are strategies to help you manage stress and improve your fertility journey:

- **Understand the Connection:**
  - Chronic stress can disrupt hormonal balance, affecting ovulation in women and sperm production in men.
  - Recognize that stress is a natural part of life, but chronic, unmanaged stress can be detrimental to fertility.

- **Prioritize Self-Care:**
  - Make self-care a priority. This includes activities that relax and rejuvenate you, such as meditation, deep breathing, yoga, or hobbies you enjoy.

- **Practice Mindfulness:**
  - Mindfulness meditation can help reduce stress. Spend a few minutes each day focusing on your breath and being present in the moment.

- **Maintain a Healthy Lifestyle:**
  - Eat a balanced diet, exercise regularly, and get enough sleep to support your overall health and reduce stress.

- **Seek Support:**

- Talk to your partner about your feelings and concerns. Emotional support is crucial during the fertility journey.

- Consider joining a support group or seeking counseling if you find it challenging to manage stress on your own.

- **Set Realistic Expectations:**

- Understand that fertility treatments and the journey itself can be stressful. Set realistic expectations and be patient with yourself.

- **Manage Time Wisely:**

- Organize your schedule to include time for relaxation and stress-relief activities.

- Learn to say no when necessary to avoid overcommitting.

- **Identify Stress Triggers:**

- Recognize the situations or factors that trigger stress in your life, and develop strategies to address or avoid them.

- **Exercise Regularly:**

- Moderate exercise can help reduce stress. Incorporate physical activity into your routine, but avoid excessive exercise.

- **Seek Professional Help:**

- If you find it challenging to manage stress on your own, consider seeking support from a therapist or counselor experienced in fertility-related stress.

- **Mind-Body Practices:**

- Consider mind-body practices like acupuncture, which some people find helpful for stress reduction and fertility support.

- **Be Kind to Yourself:**

- Remember that fertility is a journey with ups and downs. Be kind to yourself and acknowledge your efforts and progress.

Managing stress is not only beneficial for fertility but also for your overall well-being. By incorporating stress reduction techniques into your daily life and seeking support when needed, you can create a healthier, more balanced environment for your fertility journey.

SLEEP AND FERTILITY

Getting adequate and restful sleep is crucial for your fertility journey. Here's why sleep matters and tips to improve your sleep quality for better reproductive health:

- **The Importance of Sleep:**
- Sleep plays a vital role in regulating hormones, including those that govern the menstrual cycle in women and sperm production in men.
- Quality sleep supports overall physical and emotional well-being, which is essential for fertility.

- **Aim for 7-9 Hours:**
- Aim to get 7-9 hours of sleep per night. Consistency in your sleep schedule is important.

- **Create a Relaxing Bedtime Routine:**
- Establish a calming bedtime routine to signal to your body that it's time to wind down. This might include reading, gentle stretching, or relaxation exercises.

- **Limit Screen Time Before Bed:**
- Exposure to the blue light emitted by screens (phones, tablets, computers) can interfere with sleep. Avoid screens for at least an hour before bedtime.

- **Maintain a Comfortable Sleep Environment:**
- Ensure your sleep environment is comfortable and conducive to rest. This includes a comfortable mattress and a cool, dark room.

- **Manage Stress:**
- Stress can disrupt sleep patterns. Practice stress management techniques such as meditation, deep breathing, or progressive muscle relaxation.

- **Watch Your Diet:**
- Avoid heavy meals, caffeine, and alcohol close to bedtime. These can interfere with sleep quality.

- **Be Active During the Day:**
- Regular physical activity can promote better sleep. However, avoid intense exercise close to bedtime.

- **Manage Anxiety and Worry:**
- If racing thoughts keep you awake, consider keeping a journal to jot down your concerns before bedtime.

- **Seek Professional Help if Needed:**
- If you have persistent sleep difficulties, consider consulting a healthcare provider or sleep specialist for guidance.

- **Consider Sleep Apnea Screening:**

- Sleep apnea, a condition where breathing temporarily stops during sleep, can affect fertility. If you suspect sleep apnea, discuss it with a healthcare provider.

- **Communicate with Your Partner:**

- If you share a bed with your partner, communicate about your sleep needs and preferences to ensure both of you get adequate rest.

- **Maintain a Consistent Sleep Schedule:**

- Go to bed and wake up at the same times every day, even on weekends. Consistency helps regulate your body's internal clock.

- **Be Patient:**

- Improving sleep habits may take time. Be patient with yourself as you work toward better sleep.

Prioritizing restful sleep is a crucial aspect of supporting your fertility journey. By making sleep a priority and practicing good sleep hygiene, you can create the optimal conditions for reproductive health and overall well-being.

CHAPTER 10

SUPPORTING EACH OTHER ON THE FERTILITY JOURNEY

The fertility journey can be emotionally and physically challenging for both partners. In this chapter, we'll explore ways to strengthen your relationship and provide mutual support during this important time.

By the end of this chapter, you'll have a better understanding of how to navigate the emotional aspects of the fertility journey together. Strengthening your relationship, maintaining open communication, and providing unwavering support to each other can help you face the challenges and celebrate the successes as you work toward your goal of starting or growing your family.

COMMUNICATION TIPS

Effective communication is essential during the fertility journey. Here are some communication tips to support each other:

- **Create A Safe Space:**
  - Foster an environment where both partners feel comfortable sharing their thoughts, emotions, and concerns without judgment.

- **Listen Actively:**
- When your partner is talking, give them your full attention. Avoid interrupting and provide validation for their feelings.

- **Use "I" Statements:**
- Instead of saying, "You make me feel," say, "I feel this way." This helps to express your feelings without blaming your partner.

- **Be Empathetic:**
- Try to understand your partner's perspective and show empathy. Acknowledge their feelings, even if you don't fully comprehend them.

- **Ask Open-Ended Questions:**
- Encourage conversation by asking open-ended questions that invite your partner to share more about their thoughts and feelings.

- **Set Regular Communication Times:**
- Establish designated times to discuss your fertility journey. This helps prevent the topic from becoming overwhelming.

- **Be Patient:**

- The fertility journey can be emotionally challenging. Be patient with each other and give space when needed.

- **Share Responsibility:**

- Both partners should actively participate in decision-making and seek input from each other regarding treatments and lifestyle changes.

- **Avoid Assumptions:**

- Don't assume you know how your partner feels. Instead, ask and listen to their perspective.

- **Use Nonverbal Cues:**

- Sometimes, nonverbal cues like a hug or a reassuring touch can convey support and understanding.

- **Seek Professional Help:**

- If communication becomes difficult, consider couples therapy or counseling with a specialist in fertility-related issues.

- **Manage Conflict:**

- Disagreements are natural, but it's essential to resolve conflicts constructively. Focus on finding solutions rather than assigning blame.

- **Maintain Privacy:**

- Remember that not all family and friends need to be involved in your fertility discussions. Keep private matters between you and your partner if that's what you're comfortable with.

- **Celebrate Small Wins:**

- Acknowledge and celebrate even the smallest milestones and achievements in your journey. This can help maintain a positive outlook.

Effective communication can help you navigate the emotional ups and downs of the fertility journey and strengthen your partnership. Remember that both partners are going through this experience, and providing support and understanding can make a significant difference in the process.

EMOTIONAL SUPPORT

Emotional support is a critical aspect of the fertility journey. Both partners may experience a wide range of emotions, from hope and excitement to frustration and disappointment. Here's how to provide and receive emotional support:

- **Empathetic Listening:**

- When your partner shares their thoughts and feelings, listen with empathy. Understand that their emotions are valid and that you're there to support them.

- **Open Dialogue:**

- Encourage open and honest conversation. Create a safe space where both partners can express their emotions without judgment.

- **Share Your Own Feelings:**

- It's important to communicate your own emotions as well. Sharing your feelings can help your partner understand your perspective.

- **Be Patient:**

- Understand that the fertility journey can be emotionally draining. Be patient with each other, especially during difficult times.

- **Manage Stress Together:**

- Explore stress-reduction techniques that both partners can practice together, such as meditation, yoga, or deep breathing exercises.

- **Seek Professional Help:**

- If the emotional challenges become overwhelming, consider couples therapy or individual counseling.

Therapists with experience in fertility issues can provide guidance and support.

- **Encourage Self-Care:**
  - Remind each other to prioritize self-care. Encourage activities that bring joy and relaxation, whether it's reading, taking walks, or pursuing hobbies.

- **Celebrate Small Victories:**
  - Acknowledge and celebrate even the smallest milestones or achievements in your fertility journey. These moments can provide hope and motivation.

- **Support Decision-Making:**
  - Understand that treatment decisions can be difficult. Support each other in making choices that feel right for both of you.

- **Maintain Intimacy:**
  - Nurture physical and emotional intimacy in your relationship. Remember that you're partners in this journey, and staying close can help you navigate the challenges together.

- **Educate Yourself:**
  - Take the time to educate yourself about fertility and the treatments you're considering. Knowledge can empower you both and alleviate fears.

- **Lean on Your Support Network:**

- Reach out to friends, family, or support groups. Sharing your experiences with others who understand can be comforting.

- **Be Mindful of Triggers:**

- Recognize potential emotional triggers, such as social events or anniversaries, and be prepared to provide extra support during these times.

- **Keep the Bigger Picture in Mind:**

- Remember that the journey may be challenging, but you're working towards the goal of starting or growing your family. Keeping this perspective can provide motivation.

Emotional support is a vital part of the fertility journey. By providing understanding, patience, and a listening ear to your partner, you can navigate the emotional ups and downs together and strengthen your connection.

CHAPTER 11:

BEYOND THE COOKBOOK

In this final chapter, we explore what comes next after your journey through the "The Ultimate Fertility Diet Cookbook for Couples" It's important to recognize that your fertility journey doesn't end with a cookbook. Here, we'll address the next steps and considerations:

- **The Continuing Fertility Journey:**
  - Acknowledge that the path to conception and parenthood is unique for each couple. Understand that the journey doesn't end with the recipes in this cookbook.

- **Seek Professional Guidance:**
  - The cookbook is a resource, but fertility is a complex subject. If you haven't already, consider consulting a healthcare provider or fertility specialist for personalized guidance based on your unique situation.

- **Emotional Well-Being:**
  - Continue to prioritize your emotional health. The journey may include more challenges, and managing emotions is key.

- **Lifestyle Adjustments:**

- Stay committed to the lifestyle changes you've made. Whether it's diet, exercise, or stress management, maintaining a healthy lifestyle is important for reproductive health.

- **Stay Informed:**

- Keep up to date with the latest research and developments in the field of fertility and reproductive health.

- **Advocate for Yourself:**

- Be an advocate for your own health. If you have concerns or questions, don't hesitate to ask your healthcare provider for clarification or options.

- **Support Each Other:**

- Continue to provide emotional support to your partner. The journey may involve setbacks, and a strong partnership is crucial.

- **Explore Alternative Paths:**

- Understand that there are various paths to parenthood, including adoption and assisted reproductive technologies. Be open to exploring alternatives if necessary.

- **Building a Family:**

- Remember that a family can be built in different ways. The definition of family extends beyond biological ties.

- **Celebrate Success:**

- Regardless of the outcome of your fertility journey, celebrate your strength, resilience, and love for each other.

- **Giving Back:**

- Consider how your experiences might allow you to support others on similar journeys. Whether through mentorship, advocacy, or sharing your story, your experiences can help others.

- **Reflect and Reassess:**

- Periodically reflect on your journey and reassess your goals and priorities. Life can lead us in unexpected directions, and your path may evolve.

As you move beyond the cookbook and continue your fertility journey, remember that you're not alone. Many couples face similar challenges, and there is a supportive community ready to provide guidance and understanding. Whether your path leads to parenthood or in a different direction, the love and resilience you've demonstrated throughout your journey will remain an integral part of your story.

WHEN TO SEEK PROFESSIONAL HELP

Knowing when to seek professional help during your fertility journey is essential for timely and effective guidance. Here are some key indicators that may suggest it's time to consult a healthcare provider or fertility specialist:

- **Trying for a Year or More:**

If you're under 35 and have been actively trying to conceive for a year without success, it's a good time to seek professional guidance. If you're 35 or older, consider seeking help after six months of trying.

- **Irregular Menstrual Cycles:**

If you or your partner have irregular menstrual cycles, this may indicate an underlying issue that could affect fertility.

- **Known Medical Conditions:**

If you or your partner have known medical conditions that could impact fertility, such as polycystic ovary syndrome (PCOS), endometriosis, or male fertility issues, it's wise to consult a healthcare provider sooner rather than later.

- **Previous Pregnancy Losses:**

If you've experienced multiple miscarriages or other pregnancy complications, it's important to seek help to determine potential underlying causes.

- **Age Considerations:**

Female fertility tends to decline with age, especially after 35. If you're in this age group and trying to conceive, it's advisable to consult a specialist earlier.

- **Prolonged Challenges:**

If you've been through fertility treatments and faced prolonged challenges or multiple unsuccessful cycles, it's a sign that expert guidance may be necessary.

- **Male Infertility Concerns:**

If there are concerns about male fertility, including issues with sperm count or quality, consulting a fertility specialist is important.

- **Psychological Stress:**

If the emotional toll of the fertility journey is becoming overwhelming, consider seeing a therapist or counselor experienced in fertility issues.

- **Repeated Unprotected Intercourse:**

If you've been actively trying to conceive with regular, unprotected intercourse for an extended period without success, professional guidance can provide insights.

- **Lifestyle Challenges:**

If you're encountering challenges related to lifestyle factors, such as weight management, smoking, or alcohol consumption, a healthcare provider can offer support.

- **Unexplained Fertility Issues:**

Sometimes, couples face unexplained infertility, where no clear cause can be identified. In such cases, a fertility specialist can help explore potential solutions.

- **Desire for Information and Guidance:**

If you simply have questions or concerns about your fertility, or if you want to learn more about your options and potential next steps, don't hesitate to seek professional advice.

Remember that early consultation with a healthcare provider or fertility specialist can help identify and address potential issues promptly. Fertility treatment options are continually advancing, and the sooner you seek help, the more choices you may have. Each fertility journey is unique, so individual circumstances and challenges may vary, but professional guidance can provide clarity and support as you navigate this important path.

OTHER RESOURCES FOR FERTILITY

In addition to seeking professional help, there are several valuable resources and organizations that can provide information, support, and community for individuals and couples navigating fertility issues. Here are some resources you may find helpful:

- **Fertility Clinics and Specialists:**
- Fertility clinics and reproductive endocrinologists specialize in diagnosing and treating fertility issues. They offer a range of treatments, from fertility medications to in vitro fertilization (IVF).

- **RESOLVE: The National Infertility Association:**
- RESOLVE is a nonprofit organization that offers information, support, and advocacy for individuals and couples facing fertility challenges. They provide resources, support groups, and educational materials.

- **American Society for Reproductive Medicine (ASRM):**
- ASRM is a leading professional organization for fertility specialists and researchers. Their website offers

valuable information for both patients and healthcare providers.

- **The American Fertility Association (AFA):**
- AFA provides educational resources, support, and advocacy for those dealing with fertility issues. They also offer webinars and other educational events.

- **Fertility Preservation Resources:**
- If you're facing medical treatments that may impact your fertility, organizations like the Oncofertility Consortium provide information and support for fertility preservation.

- **Support Groups:**
- Local and online support groups can connect you with individuals who are going through similar experiences. RESOLVE and Fertility Within Reach offer lists of support groups.

- **Fertility Apps:**
- There are various mobile apps designed to help you track your menstrual cycle, ovulation, and fertility. Some also offer educational content and community forums.

- **Books and Literature:**
- Numerous books and publications are available that provide in-depth information on fertility and

reproductive health. You can find books written by medical professionals, researchers, and individuals who have gone through similar experiences.

- **Online Communities:**
- Online forums and communities like Fertility Friend, BabyCenter's fertility community, and Reddit's r/infertility subreddit can provide a space for sharing experiences, asking questions, and finding support.

- **Therapists and Counselors:**
- Therapists or counselors experienced in fertility issues can offer emotional support and coping strategies to manage the emotional aspects of your journey.

- **Financial Assistance Resources:**
- If cost is a concern, organizations like BabyQuest Foundation and The Tinina Q. Cade Foundation offer grants to help with fertility treatment expenses.

- **Alternative Medicine and Integrative Health:**
- Some individuals explore complementary and alternative approaches like acupuncture, naturopathy, and mind-body techniques to support their fertility journey.

When considering these resources, it's important to research and choose those that align with your specific needs and preferences. Fertility is a highly personal journey, and accessing a combination of professional medical guidance and emotional support from these resources can help you navigate the challenges and decisions you may face.

CONCLUSION

In conclusion, the fertility journey can be a complex and emotionally charged experience. "The Ultimate Fertility Diet Cookbook for Couples" is a comprehensive guide that covers various aspects of fertility, including understanding fertility, lifestyle choices, nutrition, emotional support, and much more. It offers a range of resources to help you and your partner navigate this important chapter of your lives.

Remember that fertility is a deeply personal and unique journey for each individual and couple. Seeking professional guidance when needed, maintaining open communication, and providing emotional support to each other are key aspects of a successful fertility journey.

No matter what path your fertility journey takes, it's important to approach it with patience, resilience, and the understanding that building a family can happen in many different ways. Your journey may include challenges, but it can also be a time of personal growth, connection, and hope.

While this cookbook provides a wealth of information, it's just one resource in a world of support and guidance available to you. The most important ingredient in your journey is the love and support you provide each other.

With that foundation, you have the strength to face any challenge and celebrate every success along the way.

Wishing you and your partner all the best on your fertility journey. May it lead to the joy of parenthood and a future filled with love and happiness.

CELEBRATING SUCCESS STORIES

Celebrating success stories in the context of fertility and family building is a wonderful way to inspire hope, support others on their journeys, and acknowledge the resilience and strength of individuals and couples. These success stories often serve as beacons of positivity and can highlight the different paths people take to achieve their dream of parenthood. Here's how to celebrate and share success stories:

- **Personal Celebration:**
- Celebrate your own successes, whether it's the moment you find out you're pregnant, the birth of your child, or the completion of a successful adoption. Take time to savor these moments and acknowledge your journey.

- **Share with Loved Ones:**
- Share your success with close friends and family. Let them join in your joy and celebrations.

- **Support Groups:**

- If you were part of a support group during your journey, consider sharing your story with the group. Your experiences can provide hope and encouragement to others who are still on their path.

- **Online Communities:**

- Consider sharing your story on online forums or communities that focus on fertility, such as social media groups, blogs, or websites dedicated to fertility success stories.

- **Writing and Blogging:**

- If you enjoy writing, you might consider starting a blog or writing articles to share your experiences, the challenges you faced, and the ultimate joy of achieving your family-building goals.

- **Advocacy:**

- Some individuals become advocates for fertility awareness and support by speaking at events, participating in fundraisers, or working with organizations dedicated to fertility issues.

- **Volunteer and Support Others:**

- Offer your time and support to others on their fertility journeys, whether as a mentor, a listener, or a friend who has "been there."

- **Media and Interviews:**

- Share your story through interviews with local or national media outlets to raise awareness about fertility challenges and successes.

- **Book or Documentary:**

- Some people choose to document their journey in a book, documentary, or other creative outlets. This can be a powerful way to inspire others and tell your unique story.

- **Fundraisers and Donations:**

- Consider participating in fundraisers or making donations to organizations that support fertility treatment and education.

- **Celebrate Milestones:**

- Celebrate the milestones in your journey, from the first positive pregnancy test to the birth of your child. Create memorable moments to mark these occasions.

Sharing success stories is not only a way to give back and inspire hope but also a way to find healing and closure after a challenging fertility journey. Your story can touch the lives of many others who may be going through similar experiences and searching for a glimmer of hope. It's a testament to the strength of the human spirit and the love that binds families together.

THE FUTURE OF YOUR FERTILITY JOURNEY
The future of your fertility journey is filled with possibilities, hope, and the potential for happiness. Here are a few key considerations for the future:

- **Flexibility and Adaptability:**
- Be open to adapting your plans and expectations. Fertility journeys often take unexpected turns, and your ability to be flexible can make the path smoother.

- **Professional Guidance:**
- Continue seeking guidance from healthcare providers and specialists. They can offer valuable insights and options as you move forward.

- **Lifestyle Choices:**
- Maintain lifestyle changes and habits that support your reproductive health. These include a balanced diet, regular exercise, and stress management.

- **Emotional Support:**
- Emotional well-being is an ongoing priority. Seek support from therapists or counselors as needed to help you manage the emotional aspects of your journey.

- **Exploring Alternatives:**

- Be open to exploring alternative paths to parenthood, such as adoption or assisted reproductive technologies, if your initial plans do not yield the desired results.

- **Educating Yourself:**

- Continue educating yourself about fertility and reproductive health. Knowledge is empowering, and it can help you make informed decisions.

- **Advocacy:**

- If you've experienced challenges, consider becoming an advocate for fertility awareness and support. Your experiences can help others on their journeys.

- **Celebrating Milestones:**

- Keep celebrating your milestones, whether it's a positive pregnancy test, the birth of a child, or the successful completion of an adoption process.

- **Resilience and Hope:**

- Cultivate resilience and maintain hope. The journey may be challenging, but the love and commitment that brought you together will continue to be your guiding force.

- **Building a Family:**

- Remember that family-building comes in various forms. Whether through biological children, adopted children, or other means, your family's future is bright.

- **Supporting Others:**

- Pay it forward by providing support and encouragement to others on their fertility journeys. Your experiences can be a source of inspiration and strength.

- **Future Dreams:**

- Continue dreaming about your family's future and all the wonderful moments you'll share. Your vision can be a motivating force as you move forward.

The future of your fertility journey is a continuation of your love story. It's marked by your ability to adapt, your resilience, and your unwavering commitment to building the family you desire. No matter where the path leads, your journey will be a testament to the strength of your love and the possibilities that lie ahead.

GLOSSARY OF TERMS

Fertility: The natural capability to conceive and have children.

Reproductive Health: The state of complete physical, mental, and social well-being concerning one's reproductive system and its functions.

Ovulation: The release of an egg from the ovaries, typically occurring midway through the menstrual cycle.

Menstrual Cycle: The monthly series of changes in a woman's body that prepares it for possible pregnancy.

Hormones: Chemical messengers produced by the endocrine glands that regulate various bodily functions, including reproduction.

Follicle: A fluid-filled sac in the ovaries containing an immature egg.

Sperm: The male reproductive cells necessary for fertilizing an egg.

Fertilization: The process of a sperm cell joining with an egg, resulting in the formation of a zygote.

Zygote: The initial cell formed when two gamete cells (sperm and egg) unite.

Infertility: The inability to conceive after one year of regular, unprotected intercourse, or after six months if the woman is over 35.

Assisted Reproductive Technology (ART): Medical procedures that aid in the achievement of pregnancy, including in vitro fertilization (IVF) and artificial insemination.

In Vitro Fertilization (IVF): A procedure in which an egg and sperm are combined in a laboratory to create an embryo, which is then transferred to the uterus.

Embryo: The early stage of development following fertilization, before it becomes a fetus.

Ovarian Reserve: The quantity and quality of a woman's remaining eggs.

Polycystic Ovary Syndrome (PCOS): A hormonal disorder causing enlarged ovaries and irregular menstrual cycles.

Endometriosis: A condition in which tissue similar to the lining of the uterus grows outside the uterus.

Omega-3 Fatty Acids: Essential fats that can help reduce inflammation and support reproductive health.

Luteinizing Hormone (LH): A hormone released by the pituitary gland that triggers ovulation.

Menopause: The natural biological process that marks the end of a woman's reproductive years.

Sperm: Male reproductive cells responsible for fertilizing the female egg.

Folate (Folic Acid): A B-vitamin important for fetal development and reducing the risk of neural tube defects.

Antioxidants: Compounds that protect cells from damage caused by free radicals, potentially improving egg and sperm quality.

Hormones: Chemical messengers produced by glands in the endocrine system that regulate various bodily functions, including the menstrual cycle and sperm production.

Menstrual Cycle: The monthly series of changes a woman's body goes through in preparation for a potential pregnancy.

Please note that this glossary provides general explanations, and individual situations may involve more specific or complex medical terminology. Consult with healthcare providers or specialists for personalized guidance.